**Environmental Health Criteria 30**

# PRINCIPLES FOR EVALUATING HEALTH RISKS TO PROGENY ASSOCIATED WITH EXPOSURE TO CHEMICALS DURING PREGNANCY

Published under the joint sponsorship of
the United Nations Environment Programme,
the International Labour Organisation,
and the World Health Organization

World Health Organization
Geneva, 1984

The **International Programme on Chemical Safety (IPCS)** is a joint venture of the United Nations Environment Programme, the International Labour Organisation, and the World Health Organization. The main objective of the IPCS is to carry out and disseminate evaluations of the effects of chemicals on human health and the quality of the environment. Supporting activities include the development of epidemiological, experimental laboratory, and risk-assessment methods that could produce internationally comparable results, and the development of manpower in the field of toxicology. Other activities carried out by IPCS include the development of know-how for coping with chemical accidents, coordination of laboratory testing and epidemiological studies, and promotion of research on the mechanisms of the biological action of chemicals.

ISBN 92 4 154090 7



PRINTED IN FINLAND

84/5990 – VAMMALA – 6200

CONTENTS

Page

Page

Page

## NOTE TO READERS OF THE CRITERIA DOCUMENTS

While every effort has been made to present information in the criteria documents as accurately as possible without unduly delaying their publication, mistakes might have occurred and are likely to occur in the future. In the interest of all users of the environmental health criteria documents, readers are kindly requested to communicate any errors found to the Manager of the International Programme on Chemical Safety, World Health Organization, Geneva, Switzerland, in order that they may be included in corrigenda, which will appear in subsequent volumes.

In addition, experts in any particular field dealt with in the criteria documents are kindly requested to make available to the WHO Secretariat any important published information that may have inadvertently been omitted and which may change the evaluation of health risks from exposure to the environmental agent under examination, so that the information may be considered in the event of updating and re-evaluation of the conclusions contained in the criteria documents.

IPCS TASK GROUP ON PRINCIPLES FOR EVALUATING HEALTH RISKS TO PROGENY ASSOCIATED WITH EXPOSURE TO CHEMICALS DURING PREGNANCY

---

Members


a,b,e Dr V.A. Alexandrov, N.N. Petrov Research Institute Oncology of the USSR Ministry of Health, Leningrad, USSR (Vice-Chairman[b,e])

b,e,f Dr E.L. Anderson, Office of Health and Environmental Assessment, RD-689, US Environmental Protection Agency (EPA), Washington, DC, USA

a,b,e Dr V.N. Anisimov, N.N. Petrov Research Institute of Oncology of the USSR Ministry of Health, Leningrad, USSR

b,c,e Professor C.L. Berry, Department of Morbid Anatomy, The London Hospital Medical College, London, Enland

e Dr C. Cortinas de Nava, Institute of Biomedical Investigations, National Autonomous Universtiy of Mexico, Mexico

a,b,c Dr R.L. Dixon, Laboratory of Reproductive and Developmental Toxicology, Department of Health and Human Services, National Institute of Environmental Health Sciences, Research Triangle Park, NC, USA (Chairman[b])

e Professor A.P. Dyban, Department of Embryology, Institute of Experimental Medicine, Leningrad, USSR

b,e Dr S. Fabro, Colombia Hospital for Women, Washington, DC, USA

b,e Dr W.G. Flamm, Division of Toxicology, Food and Drug Administration, Washington, DC, USA

b Dr S. Frankova, Institute of Psychology, Czechoslovak Academy of Sciences, Prague, Czechoslovakia

b,e Dr E. Guerrero, National Institute of Health, Bogota, Colombia

b Dr O.P. Heinonen, Public Health Laboratories, Helsinki, Finland

b,e Dr R. Jelinek, Institute of Experimental Medicine, Czechoslovak Academy of Sciences, Prague, Czechoslovakia

b,e Dr J.Ev. Jirasek, Research Institute for the Care of Mother and Child (UPMD), Prague, Czechoslovakia

b,c,e,f Dr K.S. Khera, Health Protection Branch, Department of Health and Welfare, Tunney's Pasture, Ottawa, Canada (Rapporteur)

b,e Professor E. Klika, Department of Histology, Faculty of General Medicine, Charles University, Prague, Czechoslovakia (Vice-Chairman[b])

Members (contd).

| | |
|---|---|
| e | Dr J. Kučera, Research Institute for the Care of Mother and Child (UPMD), Praque, Czechoslovakia |
| a,b | Professor V. Kusak, Institute of Experimental Medicine, Czechoslovak Academy of Sciences, Prahue, Czechoslovakia |
| b,d,e | Dr B.V. Leonov, Laboratory for Experimental Embryology, All-Union Research Institute of Obstetrics and Gynecology, Moscow, USSR |
| b | Professor M. Marois, Faculté de Médecine Saint-Antoine, Laboratoire d'Histologie, Paris, France (Vice-Chairman[b]) |
| b,e | Dr L. Martson, All-Union Scientific Research Institute of the Hygiene and Toxicology of Pesticides, Polymers, and Plastics, Kiev, USSR |
| e | Dr N. Matsumoto, Department of Public Health, Faculty of Medicine, University of Tokyo, Tokyo, Japan |
| b,e | Dr R.V. Merkurjeva, A.N. Sysin Institute of General and Community Hygiene, Academy of Medical Sciences of the USSR, Moscow, USSR |
| a,c,e, | Professor N.P. Napalkov, N.N. Petrov Research Institute of Oncology of the USSR Ministry of Health, Leningrad, USSR (Chairman[a]) |
| b,c,e,f | Professor D. Neubert, Institute of Toxicology and Embryo-Pharmacology of the Free University of Berlin, Berlin 33 (West) (Chairman[e,f]) |
| b,e | Dr A.I. Nikitin, Laboratory of Early Human Embryogenesis, Institute of Obstetrics and Gynecology of the USSR Academy of Medical Sciences, Leningrad, USSR |
| b,e | Dr A.K. Palmer, Department of Reproductive Toxicology, Huntingdon Research Laboratories, Huntingdon, England |
| b,e | Dr A. Pavlik, Institute of Physiology, Czechoslovak Academy of Sciences, Prague, Czechoslovakia |
| b,e | Dr R.M. Pratt, Experimental Teratogenesis Section, Laboratory of Reproductive and Developmental Toxicology, NIEHS, Research Triangle Park, NC, USA |
| b | Dr J.M. Rice, Laboratory Comparative Carcinogenesis, National Cancer Institute, Frederick Cancer Research Facility, Frederick, MD, USA |
| b | Dr L. Rosival, Centre of Hygiene, Research Institute of Preventive Medicine, Bratislava, Czechoslovakia |
| b,c,e | Dr L. Rossi, Institute of Oncology, Genoa, Italy |
| b | Dr Z. Rychter, Institute of Physiology, Czechoslovak Academy of Sciences, Prague, Czechoslovakia |

Members (contd).

| | |
|---|---|
| b,e | Dr J.G. Scandalios, Department of Genetics, North Carolina State University, Raleigh, NC, USA |
| b,e | Professor T.H. Shepard, Central Laboratory for Human Embryology, University of Washington, Seattle, Washington, USA (Vice-Chairman[e]) |
| a,b,c, e,f | Dr S. Tabacova, Institute of Hygiene and Occupational Health, Medical Academy, Sofia, Bulgaria (Rapporteur) |
| e | Dr H.A. Tilson, Laboratory of Behavioural and Neurological Toxicology, National Institute of Environmental Health Sciences, Research Triangle Park, NC, USA |
| b | Dr M. Vargova, Research Institute of Preventive Medicine, Bratislava, Czechoslovakia |
| b,e | Dr T. Vergieva, Institute of Hygiene and Occupational Health, Medical Academy, Sofia, Bulgaria |
| e | Dr B.R. Vitvitskaya, I.M. Sechenov First Moscow Medical Institute, Chair of Communal Hygiene, Moscow, USSR |

Secretariat

| | |
|---|---|
| a,e | Dr M.M. Buslajeva, Group of International Research Programmes, N.N. Petrov Research Institute of Oncology of the USSR Ministry of Health, Leningrad, USSR |
| a,b | Dr M. Draper, Medical Officer, International Programme on Chemical Safety, Division of Environmental Health, WHO, Geneva, Switzerland |
| e | Dr M. Gounar, Scientist, International Programme on Chemical Safety, Division of Environmental Health, WHO, Geneva, Switzerland |
| e | Dr Z.P. Grigorevskaja, Centre of International Projects, USSR State Committee for Science and Technology, Moscow, USSR |
| b | Dr V. Kodat, Department of Hygiene and Epidemiology, Ministry of Health of the Czech Socialist Republic, Prague, Czechoslovakia (National Focal Point for IPCS) |
| b,e | Dr A.I. Kucherenko, Scientific Officer, UNEP/IRPTC, Geneva, Switzerland |
| b,e,f | Dr A. Lihachev, Programme on Mechanisms of Carcinogenesis, IARC, Lyons, France |
| b | Dr M. Mercier, Manager, International Programme on Chemical Safety, Division of Environmental Health, WHO, Geneva, Switzerland |

Secretariat (contd).

| | |
|---|---|
| e | Dr M. Mikheev, Regional Officer for Workers' Health, WHO Regional Office for Europe, Copenhagen, Denmark |
| e | Dr L.A. Moustafa, IPCS Interregional Research Unit, WHO, Research Triangle Park, NC, USA |
| a,b,c, e,f | Dr J. Parizek, Scientist, International Programme on Chemical Safety, Division of Environmental Health, WHO, Geneva, Switzerland (Secretary) |
| e | Mr I.A. Rozov, Programme Support Service, Division of Public Information and Education for Health, WHO, Geneva, Switzerland |

---

a Preparatory meeting, Leningrad, 28-30 June 1981.
b First Task Group meeting, Prague, 30 November - 4 December 1981.
c Steering Committee.
d Alternate for Professor N.P. Napalkov at the Steering Committee.
e Second Task Group meeting, Leningrad, 8-15 June 1983.
f Editorial Committee.

# PREFACE

This monograph was prepared by an international Task Group of experts (p. 10) from thirteen countries. The generous contributions and the personal involvement of every member of the group during successive stages of the preparation of the document are gratefully acknowledged.

The aim of the document and the plans for its development were discussed at a preparatory meeting, chaired by Professor N. P. Napalkov with Dr R.L. Dixon, as Vice-Chairman. The meeting, hosted in Leningrad on 28-30 June 1981 by the N.N. Petrov Institute of Oncology of the USSR Ministry of Health, was attended by representatives from IPCS institutions that had expressed their particular interest in the project. These included, in addition to the Petrov Institute, the Institute of Experimental Medicine, Czechoslovak Academy of Sciences, Prague, the National Institute of Environmental Health Sciences (NIEHS), Research Triangle Park, and the Institute of Hygiene and Occupational Health, Medical Academy, Sofia. It was agreed that these Institutions would prepare four background papers for the first plenary meeting of the Task Group.

The first meeting of the Task Group took place in Prague, Czechoslovakia, hosted by the Ministry of Health of the Czech Socialist Republic, on 30 November - 4 December 1981. Dr R.L. Dixon was elected Chairman of the meeting and Dr V. A. Alexandrov, Professor M. Marois, and Professor E. Klika, Vice-Chairmen. Dr K. S. Khera and Dr S. Tabacova were designated Co-rapporteurs for this and subsequent Task Group meetings. The experts identified and discussed in detail the problems to be covered in the monograph and established three working groups for further development of the draft sections dealing with prenatal and postnatal manifestations of embryotoxic effects, and with non-mammalian and in vitro tests. Professor C.L. Berry, Dr L. Rossi, and Professor D. Neubert were elected leaders of the respective working-groups. The Steering Committee, consisting of the Chairmen of the preparatory and first Task Group meetings, leaders of the working groups, and the Co-rapporteurs, co-ordinated the work of the working groups, after the first Task Group meeting, and prepared a consolidated draft, which was sent for comments to all the members of the Task Group. Comments were also received from the OECD Chemicals Division.

A revised draft was prepared by Professor C.L. Berry, with the assistance of the Steering Committee, and submitted to the Task Group before its second meeting, held in Leningrad on 8-15 June 1983. Professor D. Neubert was elected Chairman of the Leningrad meeting, Dr V. A. Alexandrov and Professor T.H. Shepard, Vice-Chairmen, and Dr K. S. Khera and Dr S. Tabacova again acted as Co-rapporteurs.

The second Task Group meeting, hosted by the Petrov Institute and the USSR Commission for UNEP, completed the document, including those sections dealing with human risk assessment (on the basis of a draft prepared by Dr R.L. Dixon and Professor D. Neubert), the conclusions and recommendations of the Task Group, and explanation of terms used in the document. A small Editorial Committee consisting of Professor D. Neubert, Chairman, Dr E.L. Anderson, leader of the working group responsible at the Leningrad meeting for the human risk assessment section, and both Co-rapporteurs, was designated by the Task Group to finalize the document.

The International Programme on Chemical Safety would like to express deep gratitude to all the members of the Task Group for their work.

# 1. INTRODUCTION

This document is intended to aid in the design and assessment of studies concerned with exploring the association between exposure to chemicals during pregnancy and defective development. Personal tragedies are involved when defects are present at birth or appear later in life and the need for improved methods for the detection of embryo/fetal toxic agents, the assessment of health risks, and the prevention of unfavourable outcomes of pregnancy, is evident.

It is not possible, at the moment, to give a precise estimate of the extent to which chemicals contribute to the induction of abnormalities in human development. Though hundreds of chemicals, which have been listed by Shepard (1983), have induced embryotoxic effects in laboratory animals, very few have been shown to be teratogenic (for definition see section 9) in human beings. Differences between animals and man in metabolism, inherent sensitivity, and levels of exposure may be responsible for this apparent discrepancy. Among the problems involved in conducting epidemiological studies is the detection of chemically-induced anomalies against a background of sporadic defects. The size of an epidemiological study necessary to detect changes in the rates of some abnormalities, is so great that such studies are seldom conducted. Smaller studies may result in inaccurate risk estimates.

There are many difficulties involved in extrapolating human risk from animal studies. For example, if a chemical, tested in animals at high doses, alters maternal homeostasis, it is possible that the conclusions drawn will be inappropriate for human beings exposed to lower levels of the same chemical and that such studies may over-predict the incidence of teratogenic events.

Gross structural defects are an obvious area of concern. However, in recent years, it has become clear that consideration of developmental toxicity following prenatal exposure must be expanded to include chemically-induced embryolethality, reduced fetal growth, and functional alterations that may not be expressed until late after delivery. Some chemicals may decrease fertility by causing a loss of the early conceptus, even before pregnancy is suspected.

The processes of cellular and morphogenetic differentiation, though poorly understood, offer many potential targets for toxic chemicals. The chemicals that can alter these processes have the potential to induce adverse developmental effects. Thus, increased understanding of the underlying processes will aid in using laboratory studies to identify potential human health effects and to quantitatively estimate risks resulting from exposure to chemicals.

Current test methods are generally carried out using whole animals. Although the number of animals tested might be reduced and the studies designed more efficiently, there is no substitute for animal tests, at present. In the future, the potential of biochemical, cellular, and other in vitro approaches might be more effectively exploited.

This document includes a description of the use of laboratory data in defining the potential embryotoxic hazards of chemicals and methods of assessing the human risks associated with occupational or environmental exposure to such chemicals. Three major areas are covered including: prenatal toxic manifestations, postnatal manifestations, and short-term tests. Prenatal toxic manifestations are discussed in relation to human epidemiological studies and laboratory studies on experimental animals. In the discussion on postnatal manifestations, the emphasis is placed on test methods for the assessment of alterations in behaviour, reproduction, and of transplacental carcinogenesis following gestational chemical exposure. Short-term tests are discussed in the context of understanding the mechanisms of developmental toxicity and their potential for future application in developmental toxicity testing.

In each area, basic data and processes were considered by the Task Group in relation to three questions, i.e.,

(a) What is the value of currently used toxicity tests for predicting human risk?

(b) What are the difficulties involved in applying test results to the estimation of human health risks and hazards?

(c) How can testing strategies be improved?

The document is divided into nine sections, which differ in structure. The Introduction is followed by Section 2, which provides background information on the mechanisms of development. Section 3 is devoted to methods of assessing prenatal toxic manifestations and represents the overall views of the Working Group, in this complex field. Sections 4 and 5 include detailed discussions on postnatal events and short-term tests, respectively, since these sections present a new field and the Task Group wished to review the potential of available tests. Section 6 on human risk assessment, was considered by the Task Group to be fundamental. The Task Group's conclusions are given in Section 7 and their recommendations in Section 8. Section 9 comprises an explanation of terms used in the document.

The Task Group, aware of the existence of several guidelines published by national or international bodies (FDA, 1966, 1970; NHW, 1973; NAS, 1977; US EPA, 1978; OECD, 1981; CMEA, 1982), wish to state that the present document is not intended to replace, complement, or discuss these guidelines.

For detailed information on methods of studying prenatal toxicity, reference can be made to a number of publications including those of Nishimura et al. (1968), Shepard et al. (1975), Ebert & Marois (1976), Neubert et al. (1977b), Wilson & Fraser, (1977-78), Benesova et al. (1979), Klingberg et al. (1979), Porter & Hook (1980), and Kimmel & Buelke-Sam (1981).

This document primarily deals with chemical exposures during pregnancy and should be useful to all those concerned with the evaluation of chemical safety. Evaluation of the effects of exposure to drugs is not within the scope of this document and has been addressed in other publications (WHO, 1967; CIOMS, 1983).

There are a number of reference sources dealing with chemicals reported to be teratogenic for man and laboratory animals (Schardein, 1976; Heinonen et al., 1977; Shepard, 1983). The embryotoxic effects of chemicals are regularly assessed in the IPCS Environmental Health Criteria documents, available from the World Health Organization. The Environmental Teratology Information Center (ETIC) operated by the Oak Ridge National Laboratory (ORNL) maintains computer-stored teratological scientific literature on a large number of chemicals, listed according to CAS (Chemical Abstract Service) registry numbers. Advice on access to this information is available from the International Register of Potentially Toxic Chemicals, United Nations Environment Programme (UNEP), Geneva.

The International Clearinghouse for Birth Defects Monitoring Systems covers nineteen monitoring programmes from various countries. The results are published, annually, by the Swedish National Board of Health and Welfare, Stockholm and, quarterly, by the March of Dimes Birth Defects Foundation, White Plains, New York.

# 2. PROCESSES INVOLVED IN NORMAL AND ABNORMAL DEVELOPMENT

The purpose of this section is to give an outline so that those working in different fields can see the background against which new developments might occur. For more detailed discussions of processes involved in normal and abnormal development, see, for example, Hicks & D'Amato (1966), Thomas (1968), Langman et al. (1975), Scandalios (1979), Page et al. (1981), and Krowke & Neubert (1977).

## 2.1 Basic Events Underlying Normal Development

Embryogenesis is a finely balanced programme of cellular events, including proliferation, migration, association, differentiation, and cell death, precisely arranged to produce tissues and organs from genetic information, present in each conceptus. Underlying the morphological development of the embryo is a progressive unfolding of biochemical potentialities, determined by temporally- and spatially-regulated transcription and translation of genetic messages.

Embryogenesis involves complex interactions occurring in both time and space. In the earliest stages, rapid cell multiplication is the rule. The cells of the early embryo have vast developmental potential, depending on their relative positions in the embryonic mass. The development of primordial tissue depends strongly on the interactions of adjacent cell groups, apparently mediated by endogenous chemicals or growth modifiers. Complex processes of cell migration, pattern formation, and the penetration of one cell group by another, characterize the later stages of organogenesis (Johnston & Pratt, 1975). Final morphological and functional development occurs at different times in different species and is sometimes completed after birth.

### 2.1.1 DNA and chromosomes

DNA is the target of several mutagenic, growth-inhibiting, and carcinogenic chemicals. The eukaryotic chromosome is a complex structure mainly composed of DNA and protein (Lewin, 1980). A large part of the chromosomal protein is made up of a small group of basic proteins known collectively as histones, which may be important in controlling the functional state of DNA. All eukaryotic cells contain essentially the same types of histones. A chromatin fibre contains a double strand of DNA and associated proteins. Between cell divisions, chromatin is normally dispersed. Most chromatin can undergo the transition between dispersed (euchromatic) and condensed (heterochromatic) states. The information encoded in DNA is transferred by a multistage process to RNA (see below).

The amount of a particular mRNA, and hence the rate of specific protein synthesis, can be regulated by controlling the number of genes specific for its production. Gene amplification is one means by which a cell can produce large quantities of a specific gene product.

Microscopically visible excesses, deficiencies, or rearrangement of chromosomes and chromatids, occurring "spontaneously" or induced by chemicals, have been found to be associated with human developmental defects. Similar cytogenetic changes may result from viral infections or irradiation. Many cytotoxic agents act by inhibiting the synthesis of DNA, thereby slowing or preventing mitosis. Other chemicals interfere with the polymerization of tubulin into the microtubules of the spindles, which prevents cell division by arresting the formation of the mitotic spindle.

### 2.1.2 Transcriptional control

Each of the two steps (transcription and translation) involved in the synthesis of a protein is controlled. In eukaryotic cells, transcription occurs in the nucleus and translation outside the nucleus. These processes may also occur in mitochondria. Differential gene activation or transcriptional control is the principal mechanism for gene control in prokaryotic cells. The finding that three distinct forms of RNA polymerase (EC 2.7.7.6) are present in eukaryotic cells, transcribing different sets of genes, points to transcriptional control as a predominant mechanism regulating gene expression in eukaryotic cells.

Transcriptional controls are well documented for highly specialized single-copy genes, the products of which make up a large proportion of cellular mRNA and protein. Examples are genes for globin, ovalbumin, and metallothionein.

Eukaryotic genes seem to be transcribed from large regions of DNA, producing RNAs with up to about 20 000 nucleotides, which are then processed into smaller mRNAs, before leaving the nucleus. The process is not a conservative one, however, for a considerable fraction of the RNA is degraded, without ever leaving the nucleus. This degraded RNA represents linkage regions between structural genes. The extent of gene expression emerges as the controlling factor in differentiation, as different gene products are produced at specific developmental stages or in response to hormones.

### 2.1.3 Translational control

The generally long lifetime of eukaryotic mRNA might imply that translational control is especially important; merely turning off a gene does not stop the synthesis of its enzyme, as long as the appropriate mRNA is intact and available for translation.

The translation of mRNA after the fertilization of an oocyte is an example of translational control that seems to involve activation of a stable mRNA. The advantage of translational control is the speed with which protein synthesis can be turned on and off. The longer an mRNA can survive intact, the more important it becomes in controlling the rate of its translation. The lifetimes of mRNAs are highly variable. Enzymes that increase or decrease in quantity in response to external signals have mRNA with shorter lifetimes than enzymes that are not closely regulated. The half-lives of most mRNAs in eukaryotic cells range from about an hour to several days. The extreme case of stability of mRNA is found in an unfertilized egg, in which masked mRNA may remain untranslated for very long periods, even years, until fertilization occurs.

The amount of translation of a given message can be controlled by regulating the lifetime of the mRNA. However, little is known of the reason why some mRNAs are more stable than others or how exogenous chemicals affect this stability. Complementary sequences within the same mRNA molecule result in a specific folding, consisting of loops and hairpins. An alternative scheme suggests that the number of times some mRNAs are translated, is predetermined.

### 2.1.4 Post-translational control and significance of membrane proteins

Post-translational control involves the modification of synthesized proteins (e.g., sub unit interactions, compartmentation, turnover, conjugation of prosthetic groups, etc.).

The plasma membrane of eukaryotic cells is composed of lipid glycoproteins. Controlled membrane permeability is essential to cell maintenance and survival. The plasma membrane also serves as a site for receptors with a high affinity for specific hormones. Interactions of hormones with receptors trigger the chain of molecular events necessary for gene expression and protein synthesis. Furthermore, plasma membranes provide cell-specific antigens, and differentiated cells within an organ provide organ-specific antigens. Antigenic specificity is essential for the cell recognition required in morphogenesis and embryogenesis. Therefore, any alteration of plasma membranes by toxic chemicals can be expected to alter permeability, receptors, and immunological cell specificity, both qualitatively and quantitatively, as well as cell-cell interactions.

### 2.1.5 Placentation

The placenta is a temporary organ that establishes a functional union between mother and fetus. This unique organ transfers all the nutrients needed for development, eliminates fetal metabolic waste, synthesizes hormones essential to pregnancy, and carries out many other anabolic and catabolic functions. Placental morphology varies with species and with the stage of fetal development.

During and immediately after implantation, before the placenta has developed, the embryo depends on histiotrophic nutrition, consisting of digested endometrial cells mixed with a secretion of the endometrial glands. The histiotrophic material resorbed by the trophoblast reaches the embryonal anlage by diffusion. Another source of early embryonal nutrition is the content of the yolk sac. In mammals, the significance of the yolk sac varies considerably. It usually functions as a non-selective structure allowing transfer to the fetus of most chemicals resorbed by the trophoblast from the chorion and chorionic cavity until allantoic (embryochorionic, feto-placental) circulation is established. The yolk sac cavity, enclosed by endodermal cells and visceral mesoderm, is of nutritional importance for the embryo for up to 9 1/2 days in the hamster (Boyer, 1953), up to 10 days in the rat, and for approximately one month in man (Langman, 1969). Though its role becomes less significant with the progress of pregnancy, the yolk sac in the rabbit and rodent species continues to function in the maternal-fetal transfer of chemicals until later in pregnancy (Lambson, 1966; Seibel, 1974), when the yolk sac is separated from the gut.

The embryonal yolk sac mesoderm is the source of the first haematopoietic tissues supplying the blood cells of the embryo-chorionic circulation. During implantation, as the trophoblast penetrates into the endometrium, maternal capillaries come into contact with the trophoblastic shell, and consequently open into the trophoblastic lacunae. As the trophoblastic shell changes into the villous chorion, maternal blood begins to circulate within the intervillous space.

The chorion is vascularized by allantoic vessels. As reported by Jirasek (1980), the human embryochorionic circulation begins about day 28-30, there being a gap of about 14 days between the time when the maternochorionic (maternal) circulation and the embryochorionic (fetal) circulation are established.

The allantois is an endodermal diverticulum from the yolk sac (later hind gut) into the connecting stalk located between the yolk sac, the amnion, and anchored to the chorion. The allantois is accompanied by umbilical vessels connecting the intraembryonal vessels with the chorionic vessels. As the amnion expands, the yolk sac duct, and the connecting stalk containing the allantois and umbilical vessels are pushed together, giving rise to the umbilical cord. After establishment of the embryochorionic circulation, embryonal tissues are nourished from the embryonal blood.

Placentation is highly species-specific with important physiological and anatomical peculiarities in different mammals. The relationships between the structure and function of placental membranes have not been satisfactorily clarified.

## 2.2 Abnormal Development

The complicated series of developmental events offers a variety of time-specific targets for toxicity. Even temporary retardation in the growth of one group of cells may have serious consequences for overall development, because each step in embryogenesis may depend on a previous one and the development of numerous tissues and organs is interrelated.

The development of an organism concerns several levels of biological organization. The targets for chemical agents occur at the molecular level; chemicals may interact with DNA, RNA, membrane constituents, enzymes, receptors, etc. It does not mean, however, that the primary events resulting from these interactions need either be specific for the cells of developing systems, or lead inevitably to some kind of embryotoxicity manifestation. In teratogenicity studies, the outcome of the primary events depends on the properties of the affected morphogenetic systems (Jelinek & Rychter, 1979). Occurrence of defects depends, in principle, on the coincidence of the critical and sensitivity periods (defined in Section 9). Some factors can cause embryonic death directly by interrupting the basic life functions of the conceptus, e.g., blood circulation.

Teratogenic research was stimulated by the observation that congenital malformations in human beings could be induced by maternal exposure to thalidomide, pelvic irradiation, or by maternal infection with rubella.

Teratogenesis, mutagenesis, or carcinogenesis may occur spontaneously or may be induced by external physical or chemical treatment.

Teratogenic mechanisms have mainly been studied in laboratory animals; human data have been obtained from either case reports or epidemiological studies. The mechanisms of action of embryotoxic agents are still poorly understood, even though rapid advances are being made. Only by increasing knowledge concerning the biochemical and biological events in normal embryogenesis can the processes of teratogenesis be better understood.

Chemicals that interfere directly with embryonic or fetal development at exposures lower than those that cause apparent maternal toxicity are most likely to be of concern. Many of the most widely-recognised embryotoxic or teratogenic chemicals meet this criterion of selective action; the difference between doses that induce malformation and doses that cause maternal death or serious intoxication, may be considerable (Khera, 1983). Embryotoxic evaluation of such chemicals requires more serious attention than evaluation of chemicals that induce toxic effects in the embryo only at doses toxic to the mother. With the latter, recognition of maternal toxicity aids in controlling the risk of embryotoxic dosages. There are cases in which both embryonic and maternal effects in experimental animals are elicited within the range of human exposure levels (for instance with alcohol or methyl mercury) and the dual danger to mother and fetus should be recognized.

Many chemicals, including teratogens, when administered at high doses or very early in embryonic development, can cause embryonal or fetal death followed by resorption or abortion of the fetus. However, substances that can kill fetuses selectively in experimental animals do not necessarily induce teratogenic effects in the survivors. The association between intrauterine death, spontaneous abortion, still birth, and congenital malformation in human beings needs to be explored further.

Although very detailed studies of the teratogenic effects of drugs have been carried out on developing mammals, birds, and other submammalian species, relatively little information is available regarding biochemical changes in the human embryo. Any knowledge of these effects is the result of limited clinical observations made some time after accidental or incidental ingestion of chemotherapeutic or other agents. As yet, there is not sufficient knowledge of the associations between the various manifestations of developmental toxicity or, more precisely, the reasons for the lack of consistency in the associations. This may partly be because information on the biochemical changes in the human embryo is lacking, thus leaving a gap in the link with the apparent final common pathway that results in a marked reduction in the number of cells, as suggested by Connors (1975), or cell products, which then fail to support either full morphogenesis or complete functional maturation.

### 2.2.1 Genetic influences

As previously mentioned, morphogenesis involves precisely coordinated interactions of cell groups. Each embryonic cell depends entirely on its genome and signals coming from the exterior. Both of these can be disturbed by chemical agents transported and transformed between entry into the maternal organism and arrival at the target cells. Thus, the response to embryotoxic agents strongly depends on embryonic and maternal genotypes.

Genetic alterations can be the result either of hereditary defects, already present in the zygote, or of an acute effect on the embryonic genome. However, the importance of somatic mutations in development is not clear. Chromosomal aberrations contribute substantially to early embryonic loss and may persist in the form of proliferation mosaics.

The mechanisms that control the timing of gene expression or repression during development and result in the orderly development of the embryo, are not understood. It is not known how the products of gene expression control development, though it is obvious that an altered gene product may affect developmental selectivity. The achondroplastic gene induces dwarfism of a particular type; abnormal meiotic divisions with the production of aneuploid cells may result in embryonic death or phenotypic anomalies such as Down's syndrome or Patau's syndrome. If the genetic defect is present in the germ cells (as with defects characterized by Mendelian inheritance such as fibrocystic disease), then it will be transmitted to future generations. However, the majority of human malformations are not inherited in this way.

The considerable variation in the susceptibility of individuals to teratogens, is well documented for animals. For example, some strains of mice are markedly more susceptible to cleft palate induction by glucocorticoids, than others. Mice, in general, are more susceptible than other species, but, results of studies with highly potent fluorinated corticosteroids indicate that it would be unwise to presume that other species including rats and primates are completely resistant to cleft palate induction. The differences in susceptibility could be related to such toxicokinetic features as the rate at which the corticosteroid is absorbed, distributed, eliminated, or transformed by the maternal animal or its rate of passage across, or biotransformation by, the placenta. The nature of the chemical's interaction within the cells and tissues of the embryo (toxicodynamics) is also an important determinant of toxicity. The basic rate of embryonic development may be important. There is evidence that the number of glucocorticoid receptors in the developing palate of sensitive mice is higher than the number found in resistant strains. However, further studies are needed to establish a cause and effect relationship.

In man, epidemiological studies on the families and relatives of the malformed children have shown evidence of the influence of genetic factors in the human response to teratogens. The pathogenetic mechanism appears to be the interaction of environmental factors with several genes. This hypothesis, the polygenic or "multi-factorial" theory, has been described in detail in the human setting by Edwards (1969) and Carter (1976). For discussion concerning other factors causing malformations see Neubert et al. (1980) and Berry (1981).

In animals, the interaction of both genetic and environmental factors determines the "liability" of a given congenital malformation to become overt. Genetic predisposition is usually due to the additive effects of many genes. Thus, the various genes regulate the expression of heritability and in doing so, are influenced by the environment.

### 2.2.2 Nutrition

Malformations can be induced experimentally by nutritional imbalance. Thus, the relationship between nutrition and human congenital malformations needs further study. Contrary to the long-held view that the fetus has first claim on available nutrients, vitamin deficiencies or a reduced availability of trace metals, such as zinc (Hurley & Shrader, 1972), appear to selectively damage the animal fetus. Teratogenic effects may be caused by deficiencies that are too slight to harm the mother and may be a reflection of the nutritional requirements of the growing fetus and its lack of stored reserves. On the other hand, general malnutrition has not been found to induce teratogenic effects.

The results of recent studies in the United Kingdom have suggested that occult vitamin deficiency may be a factor in the pathogenesis of neural tube anomalies. This finding tends to emphasize that the nutritional status of the mother is an important consideration in developmental toxicity (Smithells et al., 1982, 1983).

### 2.2.3 Critical and sensitive periods during development

It is widely accepted that the developing conceptus is particularly sensitive to toxic agents during certain periods, generally related to the development of particular organ systems or types of cells. A critical phase for the induction of structural malformations usually occurs during the period of organogenesis. In the rat, for example, this critical period extends from about day 6-15 (day of finding sperms in vaginal smear counted as first day of pregnancy) of the 22-day gestation period. In man, 20-70 days after conception is perhaps the comparable period. It may be unwise to rely absolutely on these time periods.

Before implantation, specific malformations cannot be induced in the conceptus. Malformations induced with actinomycin D or cycasin administered during the preimplantation periods are probably due to the persistance of these compounds in the maternal or fetal organism until a later stage of development.

With physical agents such as X-rays, exposure can be limited exactly to a period of seconds or minutes. However, with chemical teratogens, the situation is more complicated because of the time courses of absorption, metabolism, and excretion. In addition, the actual (proximate) teratogen may be a metabolite rather than the compound administered.

If the time in gestation, when the differentiation of a particular organ is complete, is known with certainty, then a teratogen must be present prior to or at that time, if it is to be a causative agent of malformation.

It might be thought that all chemicals operating at a particular critical time in organogenesis would induce the same pattern of abnormalities, but this is not the case. Differences between species in fetal development, toxicokinetics, and toxicodynamics account partly for this variability in response caused by interplay of critical and sensitive periods.

Other forms of developmental toxicity may have the same or different periods of peak susceptibility. For example, functional (behavioural) deficits and other latent defects may originate more commonly during the period of cellular differentiation that follows organogenesis. This susceptibility extends into the period of postnatal development to a greater or lesser extent, according to species.

### 2.2.4 Abnormalities of placental development

Certain diseases (syphilis, toxoplasmosis, or viral infections) may affect the embryo indirectly by damaging the placenta. Certain placental anomalies (placenta praevia, accreta) are associated with a relatively poor pregnancy outcome, but few cases of abnormal development, entirely due to placental causes, can be singled out (Benirschke, 1975). However, the placenta is a crucial organ in development, and abnormal fetal growth and development may be related to placental insufficiency. It is also active metabolically and, for this reason, it is important, both in the biotransformation of chemicals and in determining how chemicals are distributed between fetus and mother.

### 2.2.5 Toxicokinetics and toxicodynamics

The term toxicokinetics is used in this document to emphasize the fact that the toxicity of environmental chemicals is the subject of concern in this document.

The rates of absorption, distribution, and elimination of any chemical are interrelated and collectively determine the level and duration of the presence of the compound or its metabolites in the maternal and fetal body compartments (Mirkin & Singh, 1976). The toxicokinetics of a chemical in the maternal organism determine, to a large extent, the availability of the chemical for the embryo, though the placenta may exert modifying effects.

The kinetics of a chemical vary with species, the route of administration, length of exposure, the physiological status of the animal, etc. Differences in kinetics, especially in biotransformation, account for a considerable number of species differences in response to chemicals. It has been, and continues to be, suggested that prior performance of toxicokinetic studies would make it possible to choose the most appropriate species for toxicity testing. But toxicokinetic similarity is only one of several aspects that have to be considered in the choice of a model system.

Biological responses in tissues are initiated by an interaction between a chemical and a receptor, as, for example, interactions between enzymes and substrates, oxygen and haemoglobin, catecholamines and neuroreceptors. Agents such as pharmaceutical compounds and pesticides are often designed to compete with the natural substance for the receptor or to prevent a response by altering or blocking the receptor. This process may be labelled pharmacodynamic, if desirable, and toxicodynamic if undesirable. It is generally assumed that pharmacodynamics are similar for most species and while this may be the case for individual receptors, species- and strain-differences can arise, because of the different numbers of receptors present during development.

#### 2.2.5.1 Placental transfer

Concentration gradients and physicochemical factors, such as lipid solubility, relative molecular mass, and protein-binding, determine the rate at which chemicals cross biological membranes and also largely determine the rate of placental transport. The binding of a substantial fraction of a chemical to maternal plasma proteins will reduce the concentration gradient of free (unbound) molecules and thereby diminish the rate of their passage across the placenta. The fetal plasma protein may act as a sink for the chemical molecules after they cross the placenta; therefore, a relatively large amount of a chemical may have to be transferred, against a relatively low concentration gradient, in order to establish maternal-fetal equilibrium. If the protein-binding capacity in the fetal compartment is smaller than that in the maternal organism, the free concentration of the xenobiotic may be higher in the fetus.

Substances that are very lipid-soluble (e.g., the anaesthetic gases) diffuse across the placental membranes so rapidly that their overall rates of equilibration are probably limited only by organ blood flow. Though some steroids cross the placenta readily, their glucuronide conjugates penetrate at much slower rates. In general, the placenta does not seem to represent a barrier to chemicals with relative molecular masses of approximately 300 or less, but chemicals of higher relative molecular mass appear more slowly in fetal blood after maternal exposure, because the rate of transfer is lower. However, even substances of comparatively high relative molecular mass, such as antibody globulins, viruses, cellular pathogens, and erythrocytes, pass from the maternal circulation into the fetus.

#### 2.2.5.2 Biotransformation

A number of chemicals are biotransformed into metabolites by the enzyme systems in the mother, placenta, or fetus. The exact role of genetically-determined biotransformation enzymes in influencing the expression of teratogenicity has not been ascertained for most substances. Important enzymes, in this respect, are localized in the endoplasmic reticulum and constitute a family of cytochrome P-450-dependent mono-oxygenases. Environmental chemicals that enhance or inhibit the activities of these mono-oxygenases (and thus the rate of metabolism of certain chemicals), are referred to, respectively, as inducers or inhibitors. The inducers include phenobarbital, chlordane, DDT, polycyclic aromatic hydrocarbons, flavons, dioxins, indoles, and polyhalogenated biphenyls, many of which are combustion products, industrial chemicals, and pesticides. The inhibitors include carbon monoxide (*in vitro*), imidazole, methylene blue, aniline, amines, and some more or less specific inhibitors. The ability of chemicals to induce or inhibit the activity of the microsomal enzyme systems is an important factor to be taken into account in devising experimental protocols.

### 2.2.6 Structure-activity relationship

The invention of new pharmaceutical compounds or pesticides is based on the knowledge of chemical groups that will interfere with specific enzyme reactions or act on specific receptors. The development of new chemicals is intended to enhance the desired activity and reduce undesired effects. However, a similar strategy cannot yet be extended to developmental toxicity, since it is not possible to predict, with certainty, the effects of chemicals on developmental processes, on the basis of their structure alone.

# 3. METHODS OF ASSESSING PRENATAL TOXIC MANIFESTATIONS

## 3.1 Human Studies

Human data are considered to be of great potential value. The present casual attitude to documenting abortions and examining the products of conception is a serious handicap to acquiring knowledge concerning the influence of environmental chemicals on human development. Epidemiological studies are important for identifying environmental hazards and for providing human data as a basis for validating animal models that might predict human disease before it occurs. Therefore, well-designed studies are extremely valuable and should be encouraged.

When it is suspected that the environment is contaminated from a known or unknown source, the exposed area and population should be monitored. The chemical should be identified and the levels of exposure quantified; contamination of the soil, air, water, food, animals, and people should be assessed. Specimens from these sources should be retained for future study.Information on exposure levels and/or the body burden of exposed persons can sometimes be obtained by analysis of body fluids, such as blood, urine, or breast milk, biopsy or autopsy tissues, placental tissues, hair, or extracted teeth.

### 3.1.1 Measures of reproductive outcome

Because of the complex integrated nature of reproduction in all mammalian species, abnormal reproductive performance provides a sensitive indicator of chemical effects. Widely-used measures of reproductive performance include abortion, still birth, birth weight, and peri- or neonatal death. These measures are discussed below.

#### 3.1.1.1 Abortion

An area of concern for the Task Group was the lack of general awareness of present data on human reproductive wastage, even among those who deal with the effects of chemicals on development. In addition, the Task Group considered that the acquisition of new data in this field would be of major importance in estimating putative risks from chemicals.

"Spontaneous" or induced impairment in development often results in embryonic death during early pregnancy. A spontaneous wastage of early conceptuses (15-20% abortion rate) is documented by clinical observations of embryonic loss after implantation. However, the results of studies using the beta-HCG radioimmunoassay for detecting trophoblast differentiation and implantation, as well as observations on the development of transplanted pre-implanted human embryos, have indicated that, even in a group of women who might be expected to have good reproductive performance, more than half of early conceptuses are lost within the first weeks of gestation (Miller et al., 1980; Edmonds et al., 1982; Lopata et al., 1982).

Important in its own right, the death of the conceptus becomes even more relevant, because of its frequent association with congenital malformations. Thus, while 2.5-3% of live births show major malformation, numerous studies have shown more than 90% of conceptuses with anomalies as diverse as cebocephaly, Turner's syndrome, and neural tube defects are aborted in early pregnancy (Table 1, Berry, 1981). It is becoming clear that many abnormal embryos are aborted. In spontaneous abortions occurring in the first trimester, about 60% exhibit chromosomal aberrations, mostly trisomy, monosomy, or triploidy (Boue et al., 1975).

Nishimura (1969) reported that 3.7 - 4.7% of nearly a thousand late embryos and early fetuses obtained from surgical abortions had externally visible malformations. This relatively high background of "spontaneous" abnormalities makes it difficult to detect a small increase in the overall incidence that might be caused by a single agent.

Curetted materials of 5-12 weeks gestation were collected by Watanabe (1979) from a private hospital in Nigata city, in collaboration with attending physicians, and the chromosomes of embryonic cells and chorionic villi analysed. All of the material was taken from women whose pregnancies had been terminated for socio-economic reasons only. During May 1977, 1250 cases were analysed from which 80 chromosome abnormalities were detected, giving an incidence of 6.4%. An increased incidence was found with increasing maternal age, particularly in the occurrence of complete aneuploidy.

Table 1. Malformations in aborted fetuses and newborn

| | Prevalence per 1000 | | |
|---|---|---|---|
| Malformation | At abortion | At birth | Loss % |
| Neural tube | 13.1 | 1.0 | 92 |
| Cleft lip and palate | 24.4 | 2.7 | 89 |
| Polydactyly | 9.0 | 0.9 | 90 |
| Cyclopia and cebocephaly | 6.2 | 0.1 | 98 |

From: Nishimura (1969) and Berry (1981).

In order to ascertain the frequency of chromosome aberrations among newborn infants in Japan, Higurashi (1979) screened 12 319 newborn babies, 6382 male and 5937 females, for clinical manifestations of autosomal aberrations and for sex chromatin and sex chromosome aberrations. The incidence of chromosomal aberrations was 1/725 (0.14%) for autosomal trisomy and 1/766 (0.13%) for sex chromosome aberrations. Any potential human teratogen must be evaluated against the above background. Hereditary factors, irradiation, certain drugs and chemicals, and some viruses are all known to cause malformations. However, few data are available to define the incidence of malformations induced by them. Precise evaluation of relative risks is difficult in any group with a high background incidence of abortion and a wide variation in malformations.

#### 3.1.1.2 Still births and neonatal deaths

Though still births and neonatal deaths are well recorded in some countries, their low frequencies make them weak indicators of developmental toxicity related to environmental chemicals. Clusters can be identified and studied only by using statistical data on prenatal mortality. Studies of cohorts after exposure to a chemical may include laboratory examinations to determine the body-burden of the chemical, cytogenetic studies, and examination of tissues obtained by biopsy or at autopsy.

#### 3.1.1.3 Birth weight

Birth weight is an appealing variable for study, because it is sometimes obtainable from birth certificates and is known to be markedly affected by several factors such as cigarette-smoking during pregnancy (Abel, 1980). Certain malformations are associated with low birth weight, and a few others with high birth weight (Ciba Foundation Symposium, 1974). Some agents, such as aminopterin or methotrexate, cause low birth weight, when administered early in pregnancy (Milunsky et al., 1968). Before lower birth weight for gestational age can be associated with exposure to a chemical, alternative explanations, such as differences between cases and controls in prepregnancy weight, social class, diet, and ethnicity must be excluded. With care, birth weight can be analysed as a continuous variable. Thus, subtle effects of chemicals may be detected by differences in the mean and variance of birth weight, which would not be noticed by measuring the frequency of birth weights under a fixed value (e.g., 2.5 kg).

### 3.1.1.4 Congenital malformations

Congenital malformations are recorded to a certain extent on some birth certificates, but generally the omissions are too numerous for useful study. To be detected from registry data, a teratogen or embryotoxic chemical would, of course, have to be present in the area covered by the registry. Furthermore, the coded classification of anomalies in the registry must be of sufficient detail to reveal an excess of the particular birth defect observed; e.g., the diagnosis should be listed as "limb-reduction deformity" rather than "other skeletal anomalies". Often, the use of plain language giving accurate detail can provide more reliable information than the use of strictly scientific terms. Also, the registry staff must review its data on a regular basis to determine if clustering has occurred. If a cluster is observed, the diagnoses should be verified, and a case-control study conducted to seek the cause. Rarely, if ever, do all of these events occur in a way that would make it possible for a new teratogen to be detected from a registry.

In a geographical area where chemical contamination has occurred, surveillance for congenital malformations and other effects on development may be of value. If surveillance is deemed necessary, a full description of the malformations observed should be recorded. Photographs should be taken of patients with unusual findings, to assist in documenting the abnormality.

When a potential teratogen is studied, exposed persons should, if possible, be compared with a similar group of people who were not exposed. If circumstances prevent the selection or study of such a cohort group, internal comparisons, such as high versus low exposure, may be possible.

Another approach is to study all the children of exposed mothers in an effort to identify clustering of specific types of malformations. If a cluster is found, knowing the nature of the exposure may suggest a relationship to a particular chemical. The malformation observed should be classified according to other possible aetiologies such as infection, trauma, or heredity. For example, webbed toes in a family with a history of this disorder is obviously hereditary rather than due to environmental exposure.

There are observations that suggest that offspring vary markedly in their susceptibility to embryotoxic chemicals. This is demonstrated by the occurrence of the "fetal hydantoin syndrome" in only one of four siblings whose mother continued to take phenylhydantoin during each of her four pregnancies (Allen et al., 1980).

When classifying single and multiple malformations, each child should appear in a tabulation only once. Patterns of multiple malformation should be noted, since they may provide evidence of the time at which developmental disturbances occurred.

### 3.1.2 Prenatal diagnostic procedures

These methods can be invasive or non-invasive. The detection of malformation by these methods can only be made after conception and, since many patients and health personnel do not approve of planned termination of pregnancy, their value in the prevention of malformations is limited.

#### 3.1.2.1 Invasive intrauterine techniques

Though invasive intrauterine techniques are valuable in well-defined clinical situations for diagnosis, they are not suitable for use in population studies. Invasive techniques include: (a) amniocentesis, by which it is possible to sample the amniotic fluid and obtain fetal cells for cytogenetic studies and enzyme assays as well as fluid for chemical analysis; (b) fetoscopy by means of which the fetus can be inspected directly; (c) combined fetoscopy and biopsy or d) ultrasound guided biopsy for obtaining samples of fetal blood, skin, muscle, or other tissue (such as choriomic villi) for special analysis. These methods may be combined with molecular biological techniques in the future. Such techniques include restriction enzyme fragmentation of genomic DNA, in which altered DNA restriction sites can be detected when a large percentage of the cells have the altered genotype. Specific probes can also be derived from structural gene sequences or from highly repetitive genomic DNA sequences. cDNA probes for the globin have been used to detect defects in the structural gene regions, coding for the haemoglobin proteins. Deletion of specific globin gene fragments has been found in the case of thalassaemia. Defects have been found in genes coding for the Beta-globin protein. Some of these approaches have already been applied in clinical prenatal diagnosis.

#### 3.1.2.2 Non-invasive techniques

(a) Ultrasound investigation

(i) Visualisation

Visualisation of the conceptus is possible as early as 15-20 days after conception, and heartbeat can be detected at around 35 days. Subsequently, the conceptus can be "inspected" morphologically, its size and growth determined, and some malformations diagnosed. This is a valuable technique for determining fetal growth in the mid and final trimesters. When three or four subsequent measurements of standard variables, such as the biparietal distance, are performed around weeks 18, 22, 26, and 32, a reliable estimation of the prenatal growth is obtained. Gross abnormalities, such as anencephaly, omphalocoele, and cystic kidneys can be diagnosed long before term.

(ii) Fetal heart rate monitoring

Fetal heart rate can be determined with ultrasound, and recorded in the prenatal period with special monitors. The technique permits the follow-up of acute changes, produced when the mother has been exposed to a toxic agent.

(b) X-rays

X-rays are generally only used to confirm fetal death.

(c) Analysis of maternal blood

By measuring alpha fetoprotein (AFP) in maternal plasma, it is possible to detect certain malformations, especially CNS dysraphias, without amniocentesis. The advantages and disadvantages of maternal serum AFP monitoring are being studied in several countries.

(d) Analysis of maternal urine

Various indicators of development are found in maternal urine. Levels of HCG, or its B-subunit, monitor trophoblastic (placental) development. Levels of estriol are quantified to estimate fetal "well-being" towards the end of pregnancy. The quantity of maternal urinary estriol reflects the capacity of hydroxylation of C-19 steroids at the 16 position in the fetal adrenals and liver and of the transport of these steroids into the placenta, where they are aromatized. Improved chemical tests involving analysis of maternal urine are being developed for the detection of fetal metabolic abnormalities.

### 3.1.3 Epidemiological methods[a]

The epidemiological approach contributes to the attainment of three main goals:

(a) identification of environmental teratogens;

(b) monitoring of poor pregnancy outcome in populations exposed to chemicals; and

(c) evaluation of the usefulness of preventive measures.

The following approaches can be used to assess the toxic effects of chemicals (Tables 2 and 3).

#### 3.1.3.1 Hypothesis-generating (descriptive) studies

Descriptive studies are useful for generating a hypothesis, but, alone, they are not a means of testing an aetiological hypothesis. The main aspects considered in these studies include:

(a) Case reports

The description of cases of malformation, in which a birth defect coincides with known chemical exposure, rouses suspicion that the chemical is a potential human teratogen.

(b) Surveillance

Data collection systems for the surveillance of congenital malformations have been established at both regional and national levels, e.g., the International Clearinghouse for Birth Defects Monitoring Systems, already mentioned in section 1. The value of these monitoring activities, which should be continuous programmes with rapid reporting and periodic reviews and analyses of data, is to provide background for testing hypotheses.

In the Scandinavian countries, workers are registered according to occupation (Erickson et al., 1979; Hemminki et al., 1981). This computerized registry can be linked to the occurrence of developmental hazards such as abortions and malformations, to identify populations at risk. Once a registry has been established, such data analysis is rapid and

---

[a]See also IPCS Environmental Health Criteria 27: "Guidelines on Studies in Environmental Epidemiology" Geneva, World Health Organization (1983)

Table 2. Hypothesis-generating studies and observations

| Methods | Advantages | Limitations |
|---|---|---|
| Case report | No special resources needed; calls attention to possible potential teratogens | Relationships with causal agent cannot be established; lack of information on variables of interest |
| Surveillance registers | Documentation on background and time trends | Controls not included; information sparse; occupational exposures missing; slow; limitations on further contacts |
| Correlation studies | Useful pointers to the etiological factor; Easy to design | Non-causal correlations cannot be ruled out; confounding variables difficult to control |

relatively inexpensive. The shortcomings of this approach are that not all women go out to work and some may have been in their recorded occupation for only a short time.

With standardized records, it is possible to compare data collected over a certain period. Such a registry would be useful for the chemical industry. The technique can be supplemented by special epidemiological methods including analytical studies. These methods will produce more reliable results if population-wide surveillance systems for monitoring congenital malformations are established. The longer these systems operate, the more reliable will be the information concerning both the incidence of spontaneous malformations in a population (Kučera, 1961a,b, 1977), and more will also be known of the temporal and spatial variations in the frequency of congenital malformations (Kučera, 1971a). The occurrence of unusual malformations (Kučera, 1968); and possible environmental impacts on fetal formation (e.g., maternal occupation) can be identified (Kučera, 1968b, 1971b).

A surveillance system is generally considered to be a descriptive method, that has been formally justified and is generally accepted. However, surveillance should be regarded as an essential element in further epidemiological investigation rather than a separate entity for evaluating chemical hazard and/or the subsequent risk.

Table 3. Hypothesis-testing studies

| Type of study | Advantages | Limitations |
|---|---|---|
| Cross-sectional studies | Fast to execute; Relative low cost | No incidence rate is possible, only a prevalence rate |
| | Control of confounding variables possible | Poor for cause-effect relationships |
| Case control studies | Specific; fast to execute; inexpensive; reasonable data base; control of confounding variables possible | Difficult design; difficult interpretation; exposure data usually obtained after birth |
| Cohort studies | Exposure data prior to birth; less difficult to design and interpret; control of confounding variables possible | Large, slow to execute; expensive; less specific information; many confounding variables to be controlled |

(c) Correlation studies

Correlation studies are concerned with the pattern of distribution of any health condition or malformation, as well as variations in the occurrence of a malformation in relation to time, space, and personal characteristics, in populations with various levels of exposure to chemicals. The advantages and disadvantages of hypothesis-generating studies are summarized in Table 2.

### 3.1.3.2 Hypothesis-testing (analytical) studies

These studies help in establishing cause-effect relationships and in the estimation of their magnitude.

(a) Cross-sectional studies

The objective of cross-sectional or prevalence studies is to determine the prevalence rate of a malformation in a given population. The burden and distribution of a malformation are described and its association with a potential causal factor is determined. Often a prevalence study constitutes the first phase of a prospective study and is usually conducted on a representative sample of the population, within a short period of time, to provide an "instantaneous" image about diseased and healthy groups within that population. The population and the variables to be considered must be very well defined.

(b) Case-control studies

In case-control studies, which supplement hypothesis-generating studies, the frequency of malformations and extent of exposure to a potential teratogen are compared with those in an unaffected control group. The affected individual is the starting point, while the control group may be selected from either unaffected children or those affected with another type of malformation. The advantage of such a control group is that the so-called memory bias in pregnancies with abnormal outcomes is reduced. This approach is of great value when rare outcomes, such as a specific malformation, are examined. Case-control studies are feasible, only if previous exposure is ascertained. A major problem is lack of adequate exposure data. Other advantages and disadvantages are shown in Table 3.

(c) Cohort studies

These are prospective studies in which two or more groups of people exposed to different levels (including no exposure) of a potential teratogen are followed up, and the pregnancy outcomes recorded. The prospective method tends to be more informative about the quantitative risk associated with exposure to a potential agent, and is a very valuable method for analysing the association between exposure to chemicals and subsequent developmental effects. The value of epidemiological studies in associating environmental agents with health effects is greatly increased by carefully defining the study group and its cohort. Women of child-bearing age may be grouped according to occupational exposure, prescribed drugs, age, diseases, smoking and drinking habits, and other variables of interest, but the difficulties involved in the evaluation remain. The size of study populations is a major problem. The use of epidemiological studies for risk estimation can be improved by combining study populations from several countries, an approach used successfully in the Scandinavian countries. Other advantages and disadvantages of the method are shown in Table 3.

(d) Intervention studies

In these studies, the frequency of a specific disorder in groups where corrective measures have been applied is compared with that in controls. Intervention studies can be conclusive, if they are carefully designed and there are adequate controls.

### 3.1.3.3 Populations at special risk

As with carcinogens, most human teratogens have been identified in studies on therapeutically- or occupationally-exposed populations (Sokal & Lessmann, 1960; Shepard & Fantel, 1981). This emphasizes the necessity for identifying sub-populations at high risk of producing abnormally developed offspring.

Both men and women exposed to chemicals at the workplace should be followed up to evaluate the health of their progeny. Occupational health programmes, in particular, should include reproductive data as an index of workers' health. Special attention should be paid to pregnant women who have been exposed accidentally or over a long period to high levels of chemicals, even if they appear to be in good health.

### 3.1.3.4 Confounding and complicating factors

All of the previously described methods have their limitations, if used as the only source of data for risk assessment. Of particular interest, in the design of epidemiological studies, is the consideration of confounding variables. One of the most troublesome factors is lack of agreement about what constitutes a developmental defect. Structural defects are emphasized more than abnormalities that develop later in life. As mentioned earlier, endpoints include growth retardation, functional disorders, malformation, and death. Ascertainment of malformation is incomplete, even by the end of the first year of life, while examination for minor structural changes may be haphazard or virtually non-existent. In addition, one case of malformation could be reported several times by different medical doctors, sometimes with a different diagnosis.

The accuracy of incidence rates is further complicated by differences in the frequency of malformations known to occur in different populations. The rate for the same malformation may vary significantly according to state or country. Some of this can be attributed to ethnic differences, but probably other more subtle factors are also involved. Little is known regarding the susceptibility of women of different ethnic groups to chemicals that induce birth defects. Thus, it is difficult to extrapolate epidemiological findings from one geographical area to another.

Age and parity of the mother and sex of the offspring are variables that need to be recorded. Smoking and drinking habits may play a role with regard to induction of embryotoxic effects. Thus, many variables appear capable of influencing the rates of abnormal development. Other variables include the time and method of evaluation and the interpretation of manifestations considered to be adverse. Furthermore, no woman is exposed to only a single agent, and the effects of exposure to other environmental agents and other factors such as eating and drinking habits, drug use, , and diseases acquired during pregnancy should be taken into consideration.

#### 3.1.3.5 Statistical power

Statistical power is largely determined by the frequency of unfavourable pregnancy outcomes and the size of the population under study. To define the probability that a recently introduced chemical will double the frequency of normally observed birth defects, large numbers of mother/child pairs will have to be studied, and even larger numbers will be needed, if a specific type of relatively common abnormality (e.g., ventricular septal defect) is to be investigated. Conversely, slightly lower numbers may suffice, if an increased incidence of an extremely rare abnormality coincides with exposure to a specific agent (e.g., phocomelia and thalidomide), though, in such cases, a consensus of opinion accepting the association, usually precedes completion of formal statistical analysis.

#### 3.1.3.6 Quantifying studies

As already mentioned, the main drawback of most epidemiological studies is the lack of a quantitative assessment of exposure.

The environment contains numerous chemicals to which people are continuously exposed. It is therefore difficult to isolate an exposure to a single agent, and a dose-response relationship is rarely established. The best conditions appear to be in the use of prescribed drugs, where use, dose, and dosage regimen are recorded on the prescription. Computerized linkage between prescribed drugs and pregnancy outcome has been used to establish associations between drug exposure and pregnancy outcome (Jick et al., 1982). Occupationally-exposed groups constitute another appropriate model for observational health risk studies, in particular, if complemented by analysis of the potentially toxic chemical(s) or the metabolites in body fluids.

## 3.2 Experimental Animal Studies

Developmental toxicity studies should be designed and performed in such a way as to be compatible with other types of toxicological investigation. Designing, performing, interpreting, and extrapolating specific studies in isolation rather than as part of this wider background makes it more difficult to estimate risk from extraneous agents.

For historical rather than objective reasons, the main focus of a range of reproductive toxicity tests (section 4.3.3.1 - 4.3.3.8), necessary for investigating new chemicals, is the teratogenic study, which may be more aptly designated as a test for selective embryo/fetotoxicity. These initial investigations should not be termed "teratogenicity tests" since they aim to identify a variety of effects on the mother and developing conceptus in addition to malformations (Palmer, 1976). The tests are conducted to determine: (a) deviation in prenatal variables (resorptions, fetal deaths, fetal anomalies, and fetal weight); and (b) a minimal or no-observed-adverse-effect dose that does not induce any significant deviation from normal development. The period of administration should cover the period of organogenesis, which is usually equated with daily dosing on pregnancy days 6-15 and 6-18 for rats and rabbits, respectively. During pregnancy, maternal responses should be recorded at least daily and body weight recorded regularly; a record of food consumption may also be required. Just prior to parturition, dams should be killed, litter values (number of live and dead young, fetal weights) recorded, and fetuses examined for external, visceral, and skeletal abnormalities. There are variations employing different dosing periods and some designs allow for some litters to be reared so that offspring can be examined for postnatal manifestations of prenatal toxicity.

Basically, experimental animal studies should be subdivided into two types (Palmer, 1967): (a) studies in which an endpoint is sought with a material of uncertain potential; and (b) studies in which a defined endpoint has already been established. The latter are usually second-stage investigations that might be regarded as follow-up studies after initial tests and most of the literature published in this field deals with this type of investigation. The aims and approaches of the two types of examination are quite different (Table 4).

When used in the initial testing of materials of unknown potential, the aims and approaches of the developmental toxicity study are quite different from the subsequent study in which the activity of a known and potent agent needs to be defined. For initial testing, the main priorities are: (a) to detect the lowest dosage causing an adverse effect; and (b) to determine whether the effects on the developing conceptus are selective, occurring at doses lower than those causing maternal effects.

The purpose of an initial test is accomplished if results indicate that the probability of selective effects is unlikely. Elucidating the nature of the selective action, if

Table 4. Types of experimental animal studies

| | Initial testing | Second stage investigation |
|---|---|---|
| Aims: | To determine the lowest dosage causing any adverse embryo/fetal response | To determine optimum conditions of dosage and timing for maximizing the frequency of specific malformations or other endpoints |
| Means: | Chemicals of unknown but expectedly low terato-genic potential, adminis-tered in repeated doses to determine a broad range of possible effects | Chemicals of known or expected high embryo-toxic or teratogenic potential administered as a single dose |
| Usual results: | Low rates of malforma-tions not clearly distinguishable from control values | High rates of embryotoxic effects and malformations, clearly distinguishable from control incidences |

necessary, is reserved for second-stage studies, because, with a more precise target to investigate more appropriate studies, because, with a more precise target to investigate, more appropriate studies can be designed. The design of such secondary studies must be flexible and will vary according to circumstances, to such an extent that a general account would be inadequate. The following comments are therefore confined to initial tests.

### 3.2.1 Species

Animal studies have mainly been carried out on mice, rats, hamsters, and rabbits because of high fertility, short gestation period, ease of determining the onset of pregnancy, and economy of cost and housing of animals. Other species such as ferrets, cats, dogs, pigs, and non-human primates have also been used when toxicokinetic similarities between the test species and man or a longer gestation period was thought important (Palmer, 1978).

The suitability of a test species is determined by a multitude of factors including cost, availability, ease of handling and housing, life span, and similarity to human beings in respect of both developmental processes and toxicokinetics. However, the choice is too often based on a limited and unbalanced set of factors, for example, on the assumption that sub-human primates are more similar to man than other species, because of evolutionary and toxicokinetic factors. This reasoning is valid only when the test is used to confirm a positive response to a potent material such as thalidomide.

The use of primates in prenatal studies has frequently been advocated by various authors, stressing that these animals can be used to good effect to provide a closer approximation to the likely human response to a material with a known or strongly suspected teratogenic effect (Delahunt & Lassen, 1964). As a means of demonstrating or confirming the absence of an effect, they are impractical, even when toxicokinetic similarity to man can be defined. The reason for this deficiency is that malformations occur at a low frequency, so that to detect a ten-fold increase in malformations occurring naturally at a rate of 0.1% would require 100 or more monkeys per group. Moreover, primates tend to abort defective fetuses fairly readily, so that, particularly with monotocous species, the number of endpoints that can be used may often be restricted to the two "all or none" responses of abortion or malformation.

It can be expected that, if alternative species are used, investigators will naturally exploit species that they already use in other studies because of the valuable background data already available.

### 3.2.2 Dosages and dose levels

The selection of doses and dose regimens, and prediction concerning the types of effect most likely to occur, are difficult issues. Errors in choosing dose levels are most often made because data from other studies are not used (Palmer, 1978). Cooperation between the general toxicologist and reproductive toxicologist is essential. The usual requirement is for 3 test groups and 1 control (vehicle) group; the highest dosage should induce signs of minimal maternal toxicity. It is rarely necessary to use more than 3 dose levels of a test compound, when it is administered during organogenesis to females of 2 (or more) mammalian species via a route similar to that in human exposure.

Very high doses may alter the toxicokinetics. An effective alternative is to use a single "limit" dose (equivalent to a high dosage) for chemicals with low toxicity. The high dose is best arrived at following a preliminary study in which females of the same strain and species are administered the same dose of the test material, with the same dosage regimen under conditions similar to those to be used for the main study (Palmer, 1978). Conversely, with many industrial chemicals, food additives, and pesticides, as well as materials administered by unusual routes, it may be impractical to seek a maternally toxic dose. Under these circumstances, the maximum practical dosage or a limit dosage is usually employed. The extent to which the vehicle affects absorption of the test compound or to which it could exert an independent toxic effect on the fetus or dam should be known.

### 3.2.3 Positive control groups

Inclusion of a group of animals dosed with a known teratogen is sometimes recommended. However, it would be better to use these animals for increasing the size of test groups or a negative control group rather than for creating a positive control group.

### 3.2.4 Historical controls

Control values should be collected and permanently recorded. They provide qualitative assurance of the nature of spontaneous malformations that occur in control populations. Such records also monitor the ability of the investigator to detect various subtle structural changes that occur in a variety of organ systems (Palmer, 1977b).

Historical control values for spontaneous abnormalities are difficult to use in assessing the relevance of test group observations, because they show marked temporal fluctuations and clustering, particularly for malformations, anomalies, and variants (John et al., 1982). Thus, it is often more appropriate to express historical values in terms of different blocks denoting the frequency of various effects in control groups of different average size. However, extensive historical control observations may be of value in the case of very rare (low frequency) malformations.

### 3.2.5 Dosing regimen

As mentioned, the dosing regimen employed is usually daily from days 6 to 15 of pregnancy in studies on rats, and from days 6 to 18, in studies on rabbits. The day of mating or of finding spermatozoa in vaginal smears is designated as day 0 of pregnancy. For routine testing, specified dosing periods need not be considered sacrosanct; as long as the dosing period includes the entire duration of organogenesis. The dosing periods selected represent a compromise between a short period of exposure (one day or less), which with a potent agent will usually provoke a specific response, and a longer dosing period which, because it covers a greater number of potential responses, induces a less precise response. When testing agents of unknown toxic potential, the latter is recommended as a first step.

Sometimes, the test agent may be administered more than once a day, if, for example, the results of toxicokinetic studies indicate that it has an extremely short half-life. Minipumps have been used to maintain constant blood levels (Nau et al., 1981). Conversely, for materials with a long half-life, a dosing interval of more than one day might be needed to avoid accumulation of the agent in the animal. Appropriate intervals should be based on the biological half-life of the compound.

Two or more complementary studies, each employing a short overall dosing period of 4 or 5 days, should be considered when testing compounds with either pronounced cumulative toxicity or ability to induce tolerance associated with enzyme induction or inhibition. Such refinement of the dosage regimen is particularly important, when there is only a slight margin between human exposure levels and animal test dosages (Palmer, 1978).

### 3.2.6 Route of administration

In routine tests, administration should be by the anticipated route(s) of human exposure. This is logical, since the amount and rate of a chemical that reaches the embryo varies according to the route of administration. However, it is not always true that routes allowing administration of the greatest amount of material will induce the greatest effects. For example, application of hexachlorophene to the vagina or mucous membranes results in a greater systemic reaction in mother and fetus than larger doses administered dermally or by incorporation in the diet (Thorpe, 1967; Kimmel et al., 1974).

Though administration by the intended human exposure route(s) is usually best for the prediction of the human situation, it may not always be possible to achieve other important objectives such as the administration of adequate doses or the avoidance of unnecessary stress, which in itself may induce embryo/fetal toxicity. In this respect, inhalation studies with "face only" exposure are more stressful than whole body exposure and should be used only when there is no alternative. A study in which a more practical route of administration is coupled with an awareness of species differences in toxicokinetics will often provide more meaningful data. An understanding of comparative toxicokinetics may reduce the need to examine a large number of routes of administration.

### 3.2.7 Numbers of animals and statistical analyses

Group sizes generally considered acceptable have been determined by tradition and empiricism, rather than by sound reasoning. Usually, the larger and more expensive the species, the smaller the group, in spite of the fact that, on a purely scientific basis, this can be questioned. For example, the number of primates per group should be higher than that of rabbits because the primate is monotocous and offers fewer endpoints, all of which are of an "all or none" type such as abortion or malformation. Similarly, the number of rabbits per group should be higher than that of rats, because of greater variations in the incidences of maternal and fetal death, abortion, malformations, and anomalies in the rabbit. The scientific principle holds, even though it is somewhat compensated for by the fact that it is easier to examine primate and rabbit fetuses for both visceral and skeletal anomalies.

The advantage of using polytocous species such as mice, rats, or rabbits is not because there are more sample units (litters) for analysis, but because a higher number of endpoints can be recorded and a series of responses can be obtained within litters. This makes it possible to use statistical methods, other than contingency analysis, to detect significant differences with smaller sample (group) sizes. Any comprehensive investigation of values employed in screening tests (e.g., litter size, incidences of embryonic death, malformation, anomaly, or variation) shows a litter based, non-normal distribution for which non-parametric analysis is safest (Weil, 1970; Palmer, 1974; Staples & Haseman, 1974; Haseman & Hogan, 1975; Palmer, 1976; Palmer, 1977a; Cooke, 1976, 1981; Woo & Hoar, 1979, 1982; Shirley & Hickling, 1981). There has been and remains great resistance to accepting the viewpoint that the litter, not the fetus, represents the valid sample unit and that litter values are not normally distributed.

### 3.2.8 Observations on pregnant animals

Observations on dams should include examination for signs of toxicity and regular measurement of body weight. Examination of the dam contributes to the study in two important ways: (a) by providing a reference point so that any effects on the conceptus can be judged as selective and specific, rather than secondary to toxic effects on the dam; and (b) by making it possible to ascertain whether the agent is more toxic for pregnant animals. Such a phenomenon has been observed for anti-inflammatory agents and iron dextrans (Flodh et al., 1977).

Records of food and water consumption are often requested, but rarely provide more precise information than body weights and/or clinical signs, provided dosages were correctly chosen in the first place.

In initial testing, the emphasis is logically placed on using observations on the pregnant animal to determine the selectivity of action on the conceptus. However, in second stage investigations there may be, in specific situations, a need to pay greater attention to maternal toxicity as a cause of embryo/fetal toxicity. Maternal ill-health and disease conditions in the mother have been associated with malformations in human beings (Kalter & Warkany, 1983) and toxic effects in the dam with malformations in the mouse (Khera, 1983). Thus, where exposure to chemicals at, or near, maternally toxic levels is unavoidable, greater attention should be paid to the possible consequences, for the conceptus, of maternal disorder.

### 3.2.9 Observations on the progeny

When examining the litter, fundamental requirements include the recording of the number of live young, and embryonic and fetal deaths; the number of implantations can be recorded directly or deduced. It may be useful to count corpora lutea of pregnancy (except with mice, because of the difficulty of counting) to insure against incorrectly attributing reduced litter size to treatment. With studies in which dosing is initiated at, or before implantation, or when a species, such as the pig or the sheep, that has a long gestation period is used, corpora lutea counts can contribute directly to determining embryonic loss.

Viable fetuses should be examined for external malformations, and skeletal and visceral anomalies and variations, and their sex should be determined. Other suggestions, some of which are of value while others are less useful, include:

(a) The weighing and examination of dead fetuses for abnormalities. This usually provides data that are difficult to interpret, because dead fetuses undergo decomposition.

(b) Distinguishing between early and late embryonic deaths (resorptions). This is generally a useful exercise as observations of dose-related effects can help in determining the sensitive period.

(c) The recording of individual fetal weights (or crown-rump length) of rats or mice. This is generally of little value in initial testing, unless individual fetal weight can be associated with altered fetal development, such as delayed ossification or malformation. Most investigators who record individual fetal weights rarely attempt to associate these with fetal anomalies or variations. In routine tests, it is just as effective and less tedious to weigh the entire litter and calculate the mean fetal weight. The occasional abnormal or obviously oversized or undersized fetus may be weighed individually and the result related to abnormalities.

Another disadvantage of weighing fetuses individually is that it may lead to inappropriate statistical analysis, which, in turn, would provide "statistically significant" differences between groups, which would be of little biological relevance (Palmer, 1978). Similar difficulties occur when individual crown-rump length is measured in rodents or lagomorphs. This variable is tedious to record and has little value on its own, though it may complement measurements of fetal weight and skeletal development. However, this level of effort and specificity is best reserved for second-stage studies rather than initial testing.

(d) Comparison of litter weights. This is a particularly useful parameter in initial tests, because it reflects both litter size and fetal weights. A non-specific toxic response to an agent may be seen as reduced fetal weight, at low doses, and as reduced litter size through increased deaths, at higher doses. In such circumstances, a dose-related reduction in litter weight provides useful information.

(e) The weighing of the uterus and contents (gravid uterus). Some investigators weigh the gravid uterus and subtract this from the total maternal body weight to obtain a corrected maternal body weight in the belief that this corrected weight, together with maternal weights measured during pregnancy, facilitate distinction between the maternally-mediated and direct effects of chemicals on the fetus. Other workers are not convinced that such data are enough to determine the direct effect of a chemical on the fetus.

(f) Allocation of a percentage of fetuses for either visceral or skeletal examinations. It has been suggested that 66%, 50%, or 33% of fetuses should be allocated for one or other type of examination, but this applies only to rats, mice, and hamsters. It is quite feasible to examine the fetuses of rabbits and most other species for both skeletal and visceral anomalies, thus, considerably increasing the amount of information obtained from a single study. With fetuses of the smaller species, the safest procedure is to allocate half of the fetuses in each litter for visceral examination and the other half for skeletal examination. However, the most important criterion is to ensure that sufficient fetuses and litters are examined for each technique, to make a valid statistical analysis.

Two suggested methods of visceral examination are hand sectioning (Wilson technique) and microdissection. When performed well, the Wilson technique (Wilson, 1965; Beck, 1977) is acceptable. However, good hand-sectioning is difficult to achieve and high quality is rarely attained. For the vast majority of investigators, microdissection is a safer technique for small fetuses and a better technique for large fetuses.

(g) Reporting units. Data should be reported on each endpoint in the form of a test group value (mean, median, or incidence) and an individual litter value. Reporting of malformations and anomalies should clearly indicate the specific fetuses and litters affected. Accurate interpretation and correct analysis is not possible, if anomalies are listed by type, without indicating their distribution among fetuses and litters. If developmental toxicity is recorded at dosages considerably lower than those eliciting maternal toxicity, the effect may be considered selective, and a direct effect on the embryo or a specific result of interference with its nutrition.

In concluding whether or not selective action has occurred, the answer should be positive, negative, or inconclusive. When the answer is positive or negative, the process of extrapolation can begin. When the results are inconclusive, further investigations should be carried out.

### 3.2.10 Animal husbandry and laboratory practices

Animal studies should be performed according to the highest standards of care, welfare, and husbandry, for both ethical and humane reasons. It is equally important from the practical point of view, as animals in poor condition will provide unreliable results. Furthermore, all animal studies are conducted under conditions with a large number of potential confounding variables (Chance, 1957; Biggers et al., 1958; Russell & Burch, 1959; Kalter, 1965; Laroche, 1965; Dearborn, 1967; Ellis, 1967; Kallai, 1967; Palmer, 1969). Studies involving pregnant animals may be especially susceptible to these variables because of the rapid changes in maternal physiology and in interactions between the maternal organism and the developing conceptus.

Laboratory practices necessary for scientific acceptability of any work are, honesty, care, consistency, and responsibility, in addition to those mentioned or implied in this and other sections of this report. Principles of good laboratory practice (GLP) are detailed in various regulatory requirements and presented for instance, with the guidelines mentioned in Section 1.

# 4. POSTNATAL MANIFESTATIONS

## 4.1 Introduction

The production of offspring able to adapt to postnatal life requires the development of functionally normal organs and systems. Since organs and systems may often be at greater risk of damage from the adverse effects of a chemical during the period of their development and growth, functional abnormalities in various organs and systems have at times been linked with exposure to toxic chemicals during the prenatal period. The consequences of such damage may not be readily evident, unless functional or behavioural tests are performed.

The period of organ and system maturation extends beyond the period of organogenesis and even beyond the prenatal period. Therefore, the susceptible period for the induction of insults that may lead to functional deficits is much longer than that for the induction of gross structural defects.

Functions that have been shown to be affected by prenatal and early postnatal exposure to chemicals include behaviour, reproduction, endocrine function, immune competence, xenobiotic metabolism, and various other physiological functions. Late manifestations of toxicity may include neoplasia and shortened life span.

Fetal damage by chemicals has been shown to modify enzyme ontogeny. Examples of active compounds are PCBs, TCDD, organomercurial compounds, and formaldehyde and its derivatives (Andrew & Lytz, 1981; Merkurjewa et al., 1983). Since organ-specific profiles of enzymes continue to evolve and undergo pronounced changes, long after the organs have become morphologically distinct, enzyme systems are an easy target for chemical insults. Alterations in enzyme activity indicate disturbance in the fundamental biochemical processes (Battaglia & Meschia, 1978) and in the maturation of organ functions (Stave, 1975).

It has been reported that the level of drug-metabolising microsomal monooxygenases is altered following prenatal exposure to chemical inducers, and such an effect may persist in adult life (Illsey & Lamartinière, 1979; Yanai, 1979; Salganik et al., 1980). As a result, the metabolism of chemical carcinogens, e.g., aflotoxin $B_1$, may be altered (Faris & Campbel, 1983).

Toxic agents might exert their effects by causing alterations in endocrine function and hormone levels. Hormones are the natural stimuli that evoke the synthesis of many enzymes, especially those required for adaptation to extrauterine life (Greengard, 1973; 1975a,b). Major disorders may result from impairment or imbalances in developmental endocrinology, if they occur at critical stage, when hormones normally exert discrete effects on maturation. So far, few studies have dealt with the effects of hormonally-active xenobiotics on the developmental programming processes (Illsley & Lamartinière, 1979; Lamartinière & Lucier, 1981).

Deviations in functional development may also be mediated by induced adverse effects on liver function. Prenatal rat liver does not acquire full competence until some weeks after weaning, which makes it a suitable model for studying developmental delays. There are data suggesting that in utero exposure to environmental agents may result in altered liver function (Lucier et al., 1975; Chahoud & Eggert, 1978; Lucier & McDaniel, 1979).

There are indications that compounds that interfere with adult immune systems[a] may have effects on developing immune systems (Roberts & Chapman, 1981). It has been reported that exposure to toxic substances during immune ontogenesis may induce functional defects that remain dormant until adulthood (Spyker & Fernandes, 1973), and that the stage of immune development at the time of exposure may affect the nature, magnitude, and duration of the immune defect (Pinto-Machado, 1970).

Methods of assessing organ function in progeny do not differ from those conventionally used in toxicology and are not discussed in this document. Evaluation of behaviour, reproduction, and transplacental carcinogenicity requires more specific methods and these are discussed in the following subsections. The evaluation of postnatal growth and survival has been incorporated in the subsection on behaviour (section 4.2).

## 4.2 Behaviour

The argument has been advanced that behavioural tests may be useful in the risk evaluation of prenatal exposure to chemicals, because behaviour is a functional indicator of the net sensory, motor, and integrative processes occurring in the central and peripheral nervous system (Mello, 1975). Thus, alterations in behaviour following exposure to environmental agents might be a relatively sensitive indicator of nervous system toxicity (Spyker, 1975). Because behaviour can also be influenced by the functioning of other organ systems, specific organ toxicity might also be reflected as a change in behaviour (Weiss, 1975; Tilson & Mitchell, 1980).

---

[a]Principles for assessing immunotoxic effects will be dealt with in a separate IPCS document.

Two separate phenomena underly behavioural deviations that appear as a manifestation of embryotoxicity. The first, an afferent phenomenon, involves the interaction of a chemical with a molecular entity of the developing organism, such as a receptor or a specific enzyme. The second, an efferent phenomenon, represents the consequences of this interaction at the molecular, subcellular, cellular, or cell population level. Malformations are the outcome of altered development at the cell population level and are due to disturbances in basic morphogenic processes.

An embryotoxic agent may induce behavioural deviations by:

(a) disturbing the morphogenesis of the central nervous system and consequently influencing its functional development (Langman et al., 1975; Pellegrino & Altman, 1979; Rodier et al., 1979); and

(b) affecting functional development by interfering with the processes of axogenesis, dendrogenesis, synaptogenesis, and myelination (Jacobson, 1978) or with the function of already differentiated cell populations in the brain.

The relationship between morphogenesis and functional development is far from clear. Specific components of the nervous system may be affected to induce neurobehavioural deviations, in the absence of any apparent morphological changes in the brain (Reinisch & Karow, 1977; Lundborg & Engel, 1978; Rosengarten & Friedhoff, 1979). However, this view may be too simple, since an altered rate of cell acquisition in the developing brain and other morphological changes may escape detection (Patel et al., 1977; Rodier, 1978; Bendek & Hahn, 1981). Altered structural and/or biochemical components must be present to account for functional abnormalities.

In some cases, structural defects of the central nervous system have been found not to be accompanied by behavioural changes (Brunner et al., 1978). However, the manifestations of behavioural defects may be minimized by plasticity and compensatory processes or may escape detection, because of inadequate testing.

If behavioural deviations are considered to be embryotoxic phenomena, then dose-response, stage-response, and stage-effect relationships should be demonstrated. The latter characteristics are determined by a pattern of behavioural deviations that may change in a day-to-day fashion, according to the time of chemical exposure (Rodier et al., 1979). The sensitive period for inducing behavioural deviations in animals appears broader than the period for inducing malformations of the central nervous system (Vorhees et al., 1979). Behavioural changes can be induced at certain times in the early postnatal life of mice and rats that correspond to the late prenatal and perinatal periods of human brain development (Langman et al., 1975; Lundborg & Engel, 1978; Pavlik & Jelinek, 1979; Pellegrino & Altman, 1979; Pavlik et al., 1980). The development of the human brain is characterized by intensive morphogenic and functional developmental processes during the perinatal period, which continue, even during the first and second years of life (Lewis & Patel, 1980). Thus, the relevant period of brain development in the subject must be considered in a behavioural study.

Testing procedures to be employed for assessing the mechanisms of behavioural effects should be decided on the basis of the mechanisms underlying embryotoxicity. One possible approach, may include the use of the primary interaction of chemicals with molecular entities of the developing brain, such as receptors or specific enzymes. Affinities of chemicals for the following classes of receptors could also be assessed in vitro: steroid hormone receptors, classical neurotransmitter receptors, peptidergic receptors, neuromodulator receptors. Furthermore, the rate-limiting enzymes in the synthesis and/or degradation of different mediators could be investigated. The disturbances of morphogenic and functional developmental processes that are triggered by exposure to test chemicals during brain development can also be quantified. A third approach deals with assessing behavioural functions.

### 4.2.1 Strategy of testing

Study of the behavioural effects induced by prenatal exposure to chemicals is a new field which has, so far, dealt mainly with the detection and description of behavioural deviations induced by environmental agents in experimental animals rather than with the elucidation of the mechanisms of their induction (Coyle et al., 1976; Kimmel, 1976; Rodier et al., 1979; Vorhees et al., 1979). As stated by Zbinden (1981), "there are no direct and unambiguous measures of behaviour; ... even the simplest behavioural response results from an interplay of many parts of the whole nervous system, and it is always modulated by a unique set of information stored in the memory of the experimental subject".

The incomplete knowledge of normal behaviour and its underlying mechanisms, together with the fact that the study of altered behaviour has only developed very recently, account for the lack of uniformly established and accepted strategies and methods for the evaluation of behavioural effects. No single approach or behavioural test battery has been identified as the most reliable, sensitive, and economic means of detecting behavioural disfunction following developmental insult, and, with the current state of knowledge, it is not possible to select a battery of tests from the procedures available. Thus, it is considered premature to decide on a fixed protocol to be included in routine experimental animal studies for testing chemical substances (Mitchell, 1978; Tilson & Cabe, 1978; Adams & Buelke-Sam, 1981; Zbinden, 1981).

Behavioural testing is performed after something is known about the teratological and embryotoxic effects of the agent and at exposure levels lower than those inducing structural abnormalities. It is suggested that tests be performed at two levels of sensitivity/complexity: initial and secondary. Initial testing of chemicals of unknown potential should ensure that behavioural effects are not missed. It should be broad and comprehensive with regard to the types of functions assessed. This is necessary because many types of functions may be adversely affected by an agent and these effects cannot be reliably predicted. Using test methods that monitor a number of functions simultaneously is appropriate at this stage, in order to save time, cost, and effort (Butcher, 1976; Dews & Wenger, 1979). The behavioural study should preferably be conducted in combination with a developmental toxicity study on the same progeny, so that data from the toxicity study can be used to support and clarify the behavioural findings.

Secondary testing should be performed if behavioural and/or neurological alterations are observed in initial testing, or suggested by human data, or by structure-activity relationships. More sophisticated and selective behavioural techniques, perhaps in other species, should be used to help delineate the type(s) and extent of effects produced and the possible mechanisms involved. Also, at this stage, more selective exposure regimens and testing schedules should be employed, as well as procedural controls to distinguish a direct neurotoxic action from an indirect effect. Secondary behavioural evaluations should be flexibly designed with agent specificity in mind (Adams & Buelke-Sam, 1981).

In behavioural testing, several aspects should be taken into account including the choice of functions to be assessed, the tests to be employed, the species to be used, and the factors to be controlled.

#### 4.2.1.1 Behavioural functions to be assessed

The following functional categories should be evaluated:

(a) physical growth and maturation;[a]

(b) reflex and motor functions;

(c) sensory functions;

(d) affective functions (activity/reactivity);

(e) cognitive functions (learning and memory);

(f) social behaviour; and

(g) reproductive behaviour.

Ideally, behavioural functions should be assessed as they are initiated, as well as during their development, maturation, and decline, since behavioural deficits might be expressed by: (a) retardation or abnormal development of certain functions; (b) alterations in adult function; (c) premature decline in functional capacity or induction of premature senescence (Grant, 1976). At present, most behavioural testing is done on adolescent or young adult animals, with the exception of reflex and motor development tests, which are performed in early neonatal life (Buelke-Sam & Kimmel, 1979).

#### 4.2.1.2 Tests to be used in behavioural studies

Tests used in behavioural studies are basically derived from experimental ethology, psychology, neurology, neurophysiology, and neurotoxicology. The decision regarding the tests to be used depends on several factors related to the characteristics of the animal model, the availability of technology for measuring a specific function, and on cost-effectiveness/time-efficiency factors (Tilson et al., 1980). Within a particular study, the choice of tests depends basically on the desired level of analysis. At the initial level of behavioural analysis, procedures are sought that sample a wide range of functions (e.g., apical tests), are inexpensive to perform, require little or no training of experimental animals, and make possible the assessment of large numbers of animals under study. These tests are used to provide a tentative assessment of behavioural deficits and to

---

[a] Although not behavioural parameters, physical growth and maturation are so integrated with behavioural development that they must be taken into account in any interpretation of alterations in behaviour.

quantify them as precisely as possible. However, such procedures frequently require subjective measurements, often yield quantal data, and may not be sensitive enough to detect subtle neurobehavioural perturbations.

When a more detailed evaluation is necessary, tests that require extended or special training, special behavioural instrumentation, and refined procedures are used. At this stage of analysis, behavioural tests can be supplemented with other methods to determine the mechanism(s) of action, such as neurochemical assays and sophisticated morphological examinations.

The present state of development of behavioural tests requires that these methods be validated and standardized to be maximally used in any neurobehavioural-testing programme. However, before recommending a particular testing method for routine use, it must be certain that the test actually measures the desired parameters. In this context, very few of the present behavioural test methods have been validated (Tilson et al., 1979). The choice of a test method can be greatly facilitated by knowing more about its inherent variability in normal populations. As yet, such data are scarce (Phillips et al., 1980).

Another related problem is the choice or determination of the testing sequence. In general, the testing sequence should progress from the least stressful to the more stressful procedures, for instance, from natural to manipulated behaviour (Vorhees et al., 1979). However, the possible "carry-over" effect from one test to another presents problems, for which there is no easy solution. Possibly, in initial testing, the risk of carry-over should be accepted, in order to reap the benefits of being able to correlate the responses of an individual through different procedures. If there is a suggestion of a real problem associated with carry-over, this may be resolved in second-state studies by allocating separate sub-sets of animals to each test procedure.

#### 4.2.1.3 Choice of species

The selection of suitable species obviously involves practical and economic factors. Animals with pregnancies of short duration and high fecundity are preferred. It is also important that adequate embryological, toxicological, and behavioural data are available for the species chosen. As it is preferable to study species with well-investigated normal behavioural profiles, rats and mice would be the first choice. Other species or strains may be used to investigate specific behavioural deficits only at the secondary testing level. The choice of test species at this level will greatly depend on the specific function(s) to be measured. For instance, albino rats are inappropriate for assessing visual function. The use of species that are phylogenetically close to man, such as primates, may sometimes be justified.

#### 4.2.1.4 Variables to be controlled

Control of variables is essential in behavioural studies, since the integrated and subtle nature of behaviour may make it more susceptible to factors that have little impact on other endpoints of developmental toxicity.

In the current context, this control must be exercised at the time of exposure, at the time of testing, and in between exposure and testing. The list of potential influential factors is so extensive that it cannot be dealt with adequately in this document. As brief examples, psychosocial factors such as litter size, number of animals per cage, type of cage, and frequency of contact (handling by the attendant technician or investigator) can affect performance considerably. The circadian rhythm may markedly affect performance in activity tests, so it is important not to test animals from different groups at different times of the day or night (assessment of possible effects of chemicals on circadian rythm should also be considered) (Chahoud et al., 1975).

There are pronounced maternal and litter influences operating from conception to weaning that can exert a lasting impression on maturity. Fostering and cross-fostering techniques can be applied in second-stage investigations to separate direct treatment effects from postnatal maternal influences (Spyker & Spyker, 1977). Litter size is an important factor that determines not only the level of nutrition but also the amount of social stimulation (Frankova, 1968). Variations in the litter size have been shown to affect the responses to open field and T-maze tests (Robinson, 1976; Akuta, 1979). Reducing litters to a certain standard number, in order to avoid nutritional differences, has been widely practised, but there are discrepancies in the methods of standardizing litter size for postnatal behavioural studies. However, according to some authors, standardization of litter size could introduce bias into the study (Tesh, 1977).

As in other aspects of developmental toxicity, time of exposure may be critical in the determination of the type of effect induced. Timing in the performance of behavioural tests may also be critical in the determination of the effects detected. As well as being delayed in appearance, behavioural manifestations may be multiphasic in character (Sobrian, 1977; Tabacova, 1981). Furthermore, the integrated nature of behaviour is such that the consequences of damage may be overcome by the development of adaptive or compensatory mechanisms. Ideally, therefore, behaviour should be investigated as a dynamic progression. This could be uneconomic and impractical on a routine basis, but it should be borne in mind that differences in behaviour recorded at any one time may be misleading. The research worker should also be aware that the "carry-over" effect of repeated testing may interfere with the evaluation of borderline differences.

### 4.2.2 Methods of assessment of specific functions

#### 4.2.2.1 Physical development

Growth and survival are considered to be among the most important indicators of functional normality (Wilson, 1973a; Palmer, 1976; Zbinden, 1981). From the point of view of screening, a difference in body weight gain may be a significant observation of developmental toxicity, since most physical landmarks correlate well with body weight (Adams & Buelke-Sam, 1981).

Physical development is routinely assessed by recording body weight and survival at weekly intervals from birth until weaning, as well as by registering the time of appearance of certain physical landmarks (Table 5), which should be looked for daily, starting at least one day prior to their expected appearance, until prevalent in all the test animals. However, behavioural parameters may be affected by the excessive handling of pups.

Table 5. Physical signs and the approximate time of their postnatal appearance in rats[a]

| Physical sign | Postnatal age |
|---|---|
| Pinna detachment (unfolding of external ear) | day 2 |
| Primary coat of downy hair | day 5 |
| Incisor eruption | day 8 |
| Development of fur | day 9 |
| Ear opening | day 11 |
| Eye opening | day 14 |
| Testes descent | day 25 |
| Vaginal opening | day 30 |

[a] From: Alder & Zbinden (1977).

Variations in the times of appearance listed in Table 5 can result from differences in environment, animal strain, and investigators recognition level (Hughes & Palmer, 1980). Physical development may also be influenced by the duration of pregnancy, maternal health, and litter size.

#### 4.2.2.2 Reflex development

The reflexes most frequently evaluated are the righting reflexes, negative geotaxic response, auditory startle reflex, and grasping and placing reflexes (Table 6). Variations from the quoted values can be expected. Detailed descriptions and suggested procedures for measuring these reflexes are available in the literature (Bolles & Woods, 1964; Fox, 1965; Altman & Sudarshan, 1975; Alder & Zbinden, 1977; Vergieva et al., 1981a). The normal disappearance of certain reflexes may also be important, indicating that the reflex has been integrated into more complex structures of behaviour (Lapointe & Nosal, 1979).

Table 6. Reflex development in the rat

| Test | Postnatal age of appearance[a] (mean value) |
|---|---|
| Surface righting reflex | day 1.8 |
| Negative geotaxis | day 4.8 |
| Cliff avoidance | day 4.8 |
| Palmar grasp | day 6.3 (waned) |
| Auditory startle[b] | day 11.4 |
| Vibrissae placing | day 12.5 |
| Free fall righting | day 17.5 |
| Visual placing[c] | day 17.6 |

[a] From:Smart & Dobbing (1971). For reflex ontogeny in mice, see Fox (1965).

[b] At the indicated age, the test reflects the opening of external meatus of the ear.

[c] The test may be unreliable, since the visual acuity of many albino strains is so limited that confusion with tactile (vibrissae) placing can readily occur.

### 4.2.2.3 Sensory functions

Tests to assess sensory functions are based on the localization or orientation responsiveness to stimuli. These tests are influenced by a wide range of other variables as they are based on indirect measurements (Evans, 1978). Procedures to evaluate sensory functions are simple to perform and require little investment in time and equipment, but the results are limited to quantal data (the response is scored as present or absent) and the scores are subjective (Tilson & Mitchell, 1980). Thus, these tests provide weak evidence of sensory effects. More precise details regarding the extent of the impairment require other, more sophisticated methods, based on operant conditioning (Evans, 1978; Stebbins & Rudy, 1978). However, these methods are not applicable in the pre-weaning period. The ages when specific sensory functions can be assessed are presented in Table 7. For more details concerning early sensory assessment, the reader is referred to Alder & Zbinden, (1977), Grauwiler & Leist (1977), Tesh (1977), and Zbinden, (1981).

### 4.2.2.4 Motor function

Spontaneous movements can be observed in familiar (home cage, activity cage) or unfamiliar (open field) environments, and provide information about the time of appearance and type of different motor functions. Open field studies provide more

Table 7. Specific sensory functions (rat)[a]

| Function | Postnatal age at which assessment usually starts to be possible[b] | Test |
|---|---|---|
| Vision | 18 days | pupillary reflex; visual placing response; visual cliff avoidance; |
| Hearing | 11-13 days | auditory startle[c] |
| Olfaction | 3-8 days<br>3-12 days | odour aversion<br>odour preference |
| Ultrasonic vocalization | 17-20 days | failure of vocalisation when removed from nest |

[a] Adapted from Zbinden (1981).
[b] For all these tests, different authors have established their own ranges, a practice recommended to investigators.
[c] See footnote b to Table 6.

precise data and additional information on the latency and organization of motor behaviour (Zbinden, 1981).

The procedure of normal development of spontaneous motility in rat is indicated in Table 8.

Table 8. Development of spontaneous motility in rat[a]

| Type of movement | Postnatal age of appearance |
|---|---|
| Pivoting (early ambulatory movements, showing no coordination between fore- and hindlimbs, head and pelvis) | day 1 |
| Head raising | day 8 |
| Elevation of forelimbs and shoulders | day 9 |
| Crawling substituted by walking | days 9-11 |
| Elevation of hindlimbs and pelvis | days 13-17 |

[a]From: Alder & Zbinden (1977).

In the rat, a peak of motor activity (as an integral part of overall activity) usually originates between 14 and 16 days of age and falls to adult levels at about four weeks of age (Campbell et al., 1969; Melberg et al., 1976; Randall & Campbell, 1976; Campbell & Raskin, 1978). This seems to be correlated with the concurrent development of the brainstem catecholaminergic system (Campbell & Mabry, 1973).

An open-field procedure can be used to quantify the development of motor function in the pre-weaning period. The open-field test has been successfully used in early postnatal life for detecting motor disturbances after prenatal exposure to environmental toxic substances (Kavlock et al., 1980; Tabacova et al., 1981, 1983). When used periodically during the first three postnatal weeks, disturbances in the developmental sequence of normal motor patterns can be revealed.

Another group of test methods measures movements elicited by the research worker or by some kind of mechanical device. Tests frequently employed (Table 9) assess body posture, muscle tone, motor coordination, equilibrium, and gait, and provide information on the time of appearance and achievement scores. Most of the test procedures are described in detail by Fox (1965), Altman & Sudarshan (1975), and Alder & Zbinden (1977).

Table 9. Elicited neuromuscular activities

| Activity | Reference |
|---|---|
| Hindlimb support | Alder & Abinden (1977) |
| Hanging-grip strength | Werboff et al. (1961); Altman et al. (1971) |
| Clinging to inclined plane | Cabe et al. (1978); Sobotka et al. (1974); Rivlin & Tator (1977) |
| Climbing vertical rod | Altman et al. (1971) |
| Climbing inclined screen | Werboff et al. (1962) |
| Homing response | Altman et al. (1971) |
| Crossing narrow path | Grauwiler & Leist (1977) |
| Rotating rod performance | Jones & Roberts (1968) |

Most of these tests can be performed by the end of the second and during the third postnatal week. Performance on the rotating rod is best assessed during the fourth to sixth postnatal week. The optimum time for testing may vary according to the strain of rat, the design of the rotating rod, and the operating procedure. If performed early during development, the animals have neither sufficient coordination nor strength to provide meaningful scores; if conducted too late, the individual variation may be so pronounced that intergroup comparisons are not possible. As an alternative to the rotating rod, the inclined plane test requires simpler and less expensive apparatus and can be applied over a wider age range. In the pre-weaning stages, the same apparatus can be used for assessing negative geotaxis. Generally, the inclined plane test shows less variation between individual scores and is less demanding on animals' coordination than the rotating rod.

Physical strength is assessed using activity wheels or by swimming ability. However, these tests are not practised during the pre-weaning period.

It should not be inferred that all of the tests listed must be used in the same study. A small battery of adequately chosen tests is quite sufficient for any level of analysis (Tilson et al., 1979), allows better control, and creates less disturbance for the animals.

4.2.2.5 Activity, reactivity, and emotionality

Activity is a complex measure of behaviour. It might indicate various functions of the CNS and of the whole organism, for example, motivational, affective, cognitive, and physiological responses. These various aspects of spontaneous activity demonstrate clearly the necessity for a more precise definition of what is meant by activity measurements. Prenatal exposure to toxicants may result in shifting the curve of activity development to a later period (Michaelson et al., 1974) or in producing changes in activity that disappear as the animal matures (Culver & Norton, 1976; Reiter, 1977; Tabacova et al., 1981). Longitudinal testing to uncover possible age-dependent changes in activity would therefore be advisable.

The most widely-used test for assessing activity is the open-field procedure, of which there are various modifications (Spyker et al., 1972; Grauwiler & Leist, 1977; Kavlock et al., 1980, etc.). For screening, automated methods are preferable to direct observation by the investigator (Ljungberg & Ungerstedt, 1976; Norton et al., 1976; Marsden, 1979).

Reactivity is defined as the animal's responsiveness to various external stimuli. Changes in the excitability of the nervous system can be measured experimentally as changes in overall responsiveness to environmental stimulation. Reactivity is measured as avoidance of aversive stimuli, escape responses, orienting reflexes, and startle responses. The startle response is one of the most frequently used procedures to assess the responsiveness of animals to external stimuli (Adams & Buelke-Sam, 1981). This reflex can be elicited by a variety of environmental stimuli such as auditory startle or air puff startle and has a reproducible short latency. The startle response can be influenced by changing the variables of the eliciting stimulus, the level of background stimulation, or the general responsiveness of the animal (Tilson & Mitchell, 1980). Toxicant-induced alterations in startle responsiveness can be readily interpreted, because the anatomical pathways and neurotransmitter systems that mediate this response have been reasonably well studied (Fechter, 1974; Davis, 1980). Measurement of the startle response has been highly recommended as a tool for the screening of potential neurotoxic agents (Adams & Buelke-Sam, 1981). As mentioned earlier, the startle response can also be used as a test for the development of the ear (in the preweaning period) and as a specific test for hearing.

Emotionality is directly related to spontaneous activity. In psychology, the concept persists that emotionality and exploration are inversely related. High emotionality is felt to inhibit exploration while low emotionality facilitates it. Urination and defecation in the open field are often used as criteria of emotionality (Rodier, 1978), but other criteria may also be assessed (Archer, 1973).

#### 4.2.2.6 Cognitive development

Cognitive development is essentially defined as the ability to learn or respond appropriately to a changing environment. Associative learning involves the acquisition of a response to a previously neutral stimulus, as a result of temporal association and/or reinforcement contingencies (Thompson & Glanzman, 1976). Non-associative learning is expressed by various other kinds of behaviour such as habituation, latent learning, play, and manipulation of objects.

Several experimental designs have been developed to assess associative learning in young animals (Misanin et al., 1971; Amsel et al., 1976; Blozovski & Cudennec, 1980; Gemberling et al., 1980). Although it had previously been thought that associative learning could not take place until a certain level of postnatal maturation had been reached (Campbell & Coulter, 1976), subsequent research has demonstrated associative learning in rat pups as young as 1 day old (Johanson & Hall, 1979).

Numerous methods are available for the study of learning and memory in older animals. Different kinds of learning such as simple associative learning (Pavlovian conditioning) and more complex forms of learning (such as problem solving in a Hebb-Williams maze, puzzle boxes, or tests of reasoning activity) have been studied (Rodier, 1978). The conventional criteria for learning include speed of learning, number of correct responses, and duration of latency. Data from such studies are interpreted more precisely, if behaviour in the course of learning is well analysed and spontaneous activity occurring during the testing period is carefully recorded. Analysis of the inter-trial interval on freely occurring, non-contingent responses can also provide valuable information about the presence of a neurobehavioural deficit (Frankova & Barnes, 1968).

Habituation, an example of non-associative learning, is defined as a decrease in response following repeated presentation of a stimulus. The development of habituation reflects the functional maturation of structures responsible for the development of inhibitory processes (Bronstein et al., 1974). The ontogeny of habituation has been studied by Campbell & Stehouwer (1980), who demonstrated ontogenic changes in habituation, learning, and retention during the suckling period. Methods for the assessment of learning and memory in neonatal animals have been discussed by Adams & Buelke-Sam (1981).

#### 4.2.2.7 Social behaviour

The development of social behaviour has mainly been studied in primates. Although rodents have not been used traditionally, the development of social behaviour can be assessed in this species, even during the preweaning period. The type and duration of contacts in the home cage or in a novel environment of a group (or pair) of pups can be recorded. Play activities, early sexual manifestations, and agonistic activities, are other endpoints that might prove useful (Frankova, 1973).

Social behaviour in older animals has not been used extensively to indicate developmental toxicity. Basic information on the type and characteristics of social interactions may be obtained by analysing contacts between a pair of animals of the same sex placed in the novel environment. Over 40 elements (acts and postures) have been described by Grant & Mackintosh (1963). The two most common social behaviours investigated are dominance and aggression.

Sex-dependent behaviour represents a complex set of motivationally different activities, such as courtship, pair formation, reproduction, and parental activities (Gerall & McCrady, 1970; Frankova, 1977). This category of behaviour depends on the stage of development, on environmental stimuli, as well as on the hormonal status of the organism.

### 4.2.3 Relevance of behavioural studies for human risk assessment

There is a current requirement to screen agents for developmental neurotoxicity in some countries; similar rules are also being considered in other countries. In view of the already enormous cost of safety evaluations (Johnson, 1981), great care must be taken to ensure that the studies provide meaningful information regarding potential hazard. The following requirements must be fulfilled, before routine assessment of the effects of prenatal exposure to chemicals on behaviour can be generally accepted:

(a) the test(s) should be sensitive to neurobehavioural alterations produced by a wide range of test agents or conditions;

(b) the test(s) should be standardized and validated so that accurate and reproducible results are provided within and between laboratories;

(c) the test(s) should be cost effective;

(d) the test(s) should be able to recognize chemical agents known to be neurotoxic to man.

There are several instances in which the neurobehavioural function of human progeny has been reported to be altered following <u>in utero</u> exposure to environmental agents (Tanimura, 1980). The number of examples in which there is a correspondence between observed neurobehavioural defects in human beings and effects predicted from animal studies is limited to a few agents (i.e., methylmercury, lead, psychoactive drugs). In the case of methylmercury, similar types of neurobehavioural deficits were detected in human beings and experimental animals after prenatal exposure (Reuhl & Chang, 1979).

The general lack of association reflects the need for more careful epidemiological examinations and additional basic research using animal models and agents suspected of being neurotoxic.

As developmental neurobehavioural toxicology is a recently developed field of research, not enough evidence has accumulated to convincingly demonstrate a parallel between effects in animals and human beings. Manifestation of similarities may often be obscured by inadequate testing or interpretation of data, by interspecies differences in behavioural patterns or in the plasticity of the central nervous system. Behavioural techniques have been widely used to detect and quantify neurobehavioural alterations in adult animals exposed to many environmental agents. There is good reason to believe that these techniques can also be used to assess neurobehavioural changes following prenatal exposure. The fact that the relevance of animal data to human data is less questionable in the field of adult neurotoxicity is at least partly due to the fact that more information has been accumulated in this more traditional field.

## 4.3 Reproduction

Reproduction depends on structural and functional integration of various systems. Consequently, there are many ways in which reproduction may be impaired directly or indirectly. The development of the reproductive organs takes place over a period extending beyond birth, and structural as well as functional maturation does not occur until puberty. Because of the long quiescent phase between initial formation of the basic structures and adoption of their final functional form, defects may not become apparent until a considerable time after induction, unless they are so gross as to be considered malformations. Even then, certain changes may be so extreme that they lead to incorrect determination of sex rather than to identification of a developmental error. The error is only discovered later; in man, this can be 14 - 20 years after induction.

### 4.3.1 Normal gametogenesis and development of the genital tract

In both sexes of mammalian species, the reproductive organs consist of gonads, an internal duct system, and external genitalia. Since these components arise from diverse primordia, and contributions from these primordia vary qualitatively and quantitatively in the two sexes, the development of the reproductive system is particularly complex. A detailed description of the stages of development is beyond the scope of this monograph and discussion is restricted to the stages most vulnerable to chemical action.

Primordial germ cells of both male and female, are clones of special cells present in the ectoblast at the early bilaminar stage. In later stages of development, they are transferred into the endoderm of the yolk sac. From there, the primordial germ cells migrate into the mesoblastic undifferentiated primordia of gonads located on the medioventral surface of the urogenital ridges. In individuals with normal Y chromosome expressing H-Y antigen, gonads differentiate into testes. In individuals without the Y-chromosome and H-Y antigen, the gonadal anlagen give rise to fetal ovaries. The primordial germ cells in the ovaries develop into oogonia and undergo repeated mitosis differentiating into oocytes. The latter enter meiotic prophase and become invested by granulosa cells to produce primary follicles. Thus, the oocytes in postnatal mammals are at an arrested stage of meiotic division; diffuse diplotene, dictyate, dictyotene, or resting stage (Erickson, 1967). A complete oocytic envelopment by granulosa cells separates the oocytes from the ovarian stroma.

The first meiotic metaphase is completed much later after birth shortly before ovulation. In human beings, the number of oogonia and oocytes between fetal weeks 18-22 is estimated at 5-7 million, in the newborn there are approximately 2 million oocytes, and at the age of 18-20 years about 200 000. From the whole population of human oocytes only approximately 400 undergo ovulation, assuming regular ovulation; all the others degenerate.

The embryonal testis contains testicular cords composed of primitive Sertoli cells and spermatogonia. The embryonal spermatogonia originate from the primordial germ cells while Sertoli-cells are mesodermal in origin. In the prenatal period, spermatogonia, in contact with Sertoli-cells, divide slowly by repeated mitoses, they do not differentiate into spermatocytes, and do not undergo meiosis. Spermatogenesis and the onset of meiosis in the testis follows maturation of the Sertoli-cells, a step under hormonal control (follicle-stimulating hormone (FSH), luteinizing hormone (LH), and testosterone), which begins at puberty.

Synthesis of male hormones by the fetal testis is critical for the growth and differentiation of male accessory organs during the prenatal as well as postnatal periods. The male phenotype is mainly imposed on the embryo by two types of hormones, produced in the testis, i.e., androgenic steroids and the Müllerian-inhibiting factor (MIH). Androgens, produced by Leydig cells, stimulate the development of the male reproductive ducts from the epigenital portion of the mesonephros and from the Wolfian ducts, and the development of the male external genitalia from structures located around the urogenital sinus. MIH, a non-steroid factor, produced by the embryonal testis causes the Müllerian ducts to regress. The epigenital mesonephric nephrons and Wolfian duct are forerunners of the epididymides, vasa deferentia, seminal vesicles, and ejaculatory ducts. The urogenital sinus differentiates into the urethra and gives rise to the prostate; derivatives of the genital tubercle and of the urethral plate become the penis; the labioscrotal swelling turns into the scrotum. Testosterone plays an important role in the sexual differentiation of the Central nervous system (CNS) during the perinatal period.

Testosterone is synthesized in the testis from pregnenolone. A series of steps mediated by enzymes are involved in the conversion of pregnenolone to testosterone and 5a-dihydrotestoterone, the active derivative of testosterone in some organs. Interruption of any of these steps during the critical period in pregnancy would lead to a deficiency of androgens which, in turn, might lead to the development of equivocal secondary sex characteristics (pseudohermaphroditism) with normal sex chromosomes. Thus, a decreased amount of androgen can fail to masculinize a male fetus, which might have malformed ambiguous external genitalia, hypospadia (pseudovaginal pseudoscrotal in some cases), but normal testes and the XY karyotype. In severe cases of testicular dysgenesis, if the testes fail to produce MIH, the Mullerian ducts may persist and develop into a uterus and vagina. In addition, male efferent ducts may be present in some cases.

Feminization of a male may be related to the absence of, or deficiencies in, testosterone receptors. In human males exhibiting errors in testosterone receptor, the phenotype is female despite a normal male 46,XY karyotype, and the presence of testes and regressed Müllerian ducts.

In the female, the Wolfian ducts regress and the Müllerian ducts differentiate into the oviducts, uterus, and the upper 4/5 of the vagina. The urogenital sinus gives rise to the vestibule and the lower 1/5 of the vagina, while the genital tubercle and the urethral plate develop into the clitoris and labia minora. The labioscrotal swelling turns into the labia majora. Female fetuses can be virilized or masculinized as a consequence of congenital defects in the synthesis of glucocorticoids or by the administration of androgens. In the normal female fetus, gonadal synthesis of testosterone or estrogens is not apparent and there is no evidence that the interstitial cells or follicular apparatus of the fetal ovary play any role in female genital differentiation.

In the absence of male gonadal function, the internal and external genital anlagen differentiate according to the female pattern. MIH, a protein of relatively high relative molecular mass, prevents the development of the uterus and the fallopian tubes in males. The function of testicular testosterone is (i) to stimulate the growth of the epididymis, vasa deferentia, and seminal vesicles, and (ii) to promote the stabilization/transformation of the genital sinus and urogenital tubercle, urethral plate and labioscrotal swellings into the prostate, male urethra, penis, and scrotum, respectively, and (iii) to promote the descent of the testes. Prior to the male differentiation, both the urogenital sinus and external genital anlagen acquire the capacity to convert testosterone to 5a-dihydrotestosterone (DHT) which, in these tissues, is thought to be the effective androgen (Siiteri & Wilson, 1974).

Postnatally, in both sexes, normal pituitary gonadotrophin secretion appears to be required for the maturation of germ cells and their supporting cells. The pattern of FSH and LH secretion reflects the gradual maturation of a functional hypothalamic pituitary unit, responsive to feedback inhibition by sex steroids. Sexual differences in the pattern of gonadotrophin secretion are well recognized; cyclic pulsatile in females, tonic in males.

Spermatogenesis continues throughout reproductive life. It starts with stem cells (type A spermatogonia) which, in the rat, undergo 5 mitotic divisions followed by two meiotic divisions to produce spermatids. The latter change into spermatozoa, which move to, and mature in, the epididymis.

## 4.3.2 Mechanisms of abnormal development

Adverse effects on the reproductive function of offspring, resulting from prenatal exposure to environmental chemicals, have not received sufficient attention. Examples of reproductive effects that have been related to maternal chemical exposure, are given in Table 10. Chemicals may affect either the gonadal tissues directly or antagonize the action of growth-promoting or growth inhibiting factors. However, the precise mechanisms of action are not known.

When the complexity of sexual development, gametogenesis, and reproductive tract differentiation is considered, it becomes apparent that prenatal and early postnatal chemical exposure is a special toxicological problem. The gonads, the reproductive accessory organs, and the neuroendocrine system are all vulnerable to toxicity induced by chemicals acting through unique mechanisms. The specificity of male and female developmental processes also accounts for differences in susceptibility to toxic agents between the sexes.

Dixon (1982) has recently pointed out that there are a number of periods during which the developing reproductive system is susceptible to chemical insults. Interference by xenobiotics can lead to morphological, biochemical, physiological, and/or behavioural disorders as well as to the ineffective integration of the biological processes required for successful reproductive performance. Though reduced fertility in the offspring may be the most obvious consequence of prenatal exposure to toxic environmental chemicals, more subtle effects, such as those involving secondary sexual characteristics and behaviour, are also possible.

In mammals, the female fetus is especially vulnerable to agents that damage the germ cells, because, in most species, all oocytes develop prenatally; no (or few) primordial germ cells are formed after birth. Therefore, chemicals that affect oogenesis may be expected to have a lasting effect on the fertility of the female. Particular periods of susceptibility during oogenesis with long-term toxicological effects on fertility have been shown to be connected with peak oocyte DNA synthesis periods (McLachlan & Dixon, 1973). Fetal ovaries have been reported to be a target site for the action of some environmental pollutants, particularly polycyclic aromatic hydrocarbons (MacKenzie et al., 1979a,b).

Unlike germ cell production in the mammalian female, spermatogenesis is initiated in the pubertal male, and germ cells are produced continuously throughout adulthood. Prenatal exposure to several compounds, including benzo(a)pyrene, 7,12-dimethylbenz(a)anthracene (DMBA), and diethylstilboestrol (DES), has been reported to alter male fertility (McLachlan et al., 1975; Davis et al., 1978; Gill et

Table 10. Examples of reported abnormalities of the reproductive system in the offspring of mothers treated with chemicals during pregnancy

| Type of abnormality | Species | Chemical agent | Reference |
|---|---|---|---|
| Degeneration and reduction of gonocytes in male and female fetuses | rabbit | cyclophosphamide | Gerlinger & Clavert (1964) |
| Reduced fertility in males and females | mouse | cyclophosphamide | Sotomayer & Cumming (1975) |
| Gonadal dysplasia in males and females | rat | busulfan | Forsberg & Olivecrona (1966) |
| Clitoral hypertrophy and adrenal hyperplasia in female fetuses | rat | metyrapone | Goldman (1967) |
| Decreased incidence in pregnancy and reduced litter size | rat | 2,3,7,8-tetrachloro-dibenzo-p-dioxin (TCDD) | Khera & Ruddick (1973) |
| Reduced fertility in females | mouse | procarbazine | McLachlan & Dixon (1973) |
| Reduced fertility in males and females and gonadal dysplasia | mouse | benzo(a)pyrene | Mackenzie et al. (1979a) |

al., 1979; MacKenzie et al., 1979a). Some compounds act directly on the germ cells, probably at the level of DNA, RNA, and protein synthesis; other chemicals act by interfering with the normal hormonal regulation of spermatogenesis.

Though the exact mechanisms by which chemicals can alter neuroendocrine function are not clearly understood, two possible neuroendocrine effects have been suggested that may result in impaired reproduction (McLachlan et al., 1981). The first involves an action on endogenous catecholamines which, secondarily, influences the ability of the sympathetic nervous system to stimulate gonadotrophin release; the second involves the more direct action of a chemical at specific neuroendocrine centres.

Chemicals may also affect hormone action by altering steroid synthesis, by affecting the activity of steroid-metabolizing enzymes, or by interfering with hormone-receptor interactions.

Since reproduction is a highly integrated function that involves a behavioural component, compounds that alter behaviour may result in infertile animals, even in the absence of direct toxic effects on the genital tract or the endocrine system (see section 4.2 on behaviour). Development of the integrative behaviour necessary to reproduction may be susceptible to disruption by psychotropic agents or hormonally-active xenobiotics.

Effects on reproduction may also be mediated by prenatally- or perinatally-induced disturbances in liver function. Compounds that alter the hepatic metabolism of gonadal hormones can alter the reproductive characteristics of the affected individual. The long-lasting effects of neonatal exposure to polychlorinated biphenyls (PCB) and 2,3,7,8-tetrachlorodibenzo-*p*-dioxin (TCDD) on hepatic function (Lucier et al., 1975, 1978; Lucier & McDaniel, 1979) suggest that *in utero* exposure to environmental agents may result in altered enzyme activity.

### 4.3.3 Testing procedures

A detailed discussion on methods for assessing effects of chemicals on reproductive function has recently been published by the Scientific Group on Methodologies for the Safety Evaluation of Chemicals (SGOMSEC) established jointly by WHO and SCOPE/ICSU and supported by IPCS (Vouk & Sheehan, 1983).

Potentially all of the processes in reproduction may be affected by chemicals. Fecundity tests assess spermatogenesis, sperm maturation, sperm transport, semen production, and mating, in the male, and ovulation and oviductal transport, fertilization, and implantation, in the female. These are examined collectively by measuring reproductive outcome. Results of chemically-induced reproductive failure must take into account the health of the animals after chemical exposure. When evaluating chemicals for effects on reproduction, it is critical to determine the place of observed reproductive effects within the chemical's general toxicity profile. For transplacental toxicity studies, effects on reproductive performance in offspring are most meaningful in the absence of maternal toxicity and gross malformations in the young.

Testing of chemicals for specific endpoints is likely to improve the long-term understanding of the processes affected by toxicity. This is an important area for further development. However, one of the easiest measures of reproductive capacity is the ability of male and females to mate and produce normal offsprings.

The following is an outline of a few of the reproductive tests that involve exposure to chemicals during either the prenatal or pre- and postnatal periods. Many of the comments made in section 3.2 are relevant here and will not be repeated.

#### 4.3.3.1 "Fertility test" on progeny following prenatal exposure

If a "fertility test" is to be conducted in the progeny of mice or rats following prenatal exposure, the chemical is administered over a period extending from implantation until the end of pregnancy. The progeny are allowed to litter normally and their postnatal development is observed until sexual maturity. At adulthood, the males and females of the test progeny are mated with animals that have not been previously exposed to the test chemical. All pregnant females are killed at term. Data on incidence of pregnancy, and prenatal values are evaluated for toxic effects. Up to the present, such tests have only been used for second-stage testing and have not been performed routinely. This approach is included in multigeneration studies.

#### 4.3.3.2 Multigeneration studies

There is no general agreement about the most satisfactory design for multigeneration tests or even the number of generations to be studied (Palmer, 1981). The FDA Advisory Committee (1970) reported that with a range of substances, including organophosphorus anticholinesterases, herbicides, and pesticides, adverse effects were occasionally seen after two, three, or even four generations that were not clearly evident earlier. However, it is unlikely that genuine effects would be recorded in later generations that were not evident in the first or second generations (Clegg, 1979; Leeming et al., 1982). Until recently, a minimum of two litters per generation was usually recommended, though some workers feel that the maximum possible number of litters should be obtained in one of the generations, to determine whether there is any overall effect on the maximum reproductive capacity. However, supportive data for such large studies have not been published. In some designs, some of the pregnant dams are killed in each generation so that the offspring can be examined, at term, for teratogenic effects. Some of the offspring of the third generation are subjected to full histopathological examination.

No single ideal test exists for the wide range of possible compounds that will be tested. For substances that show absolutely no adverse reproductive effects at doses up to those toxic for the parent, a two-generation, one litter per generation test, would be satisfactory. For other compounds that show a small, but increasing effect with time, more litters and more generations may be required to establish a no-observed-adverse-effect level. In practice, if only one litter is produced per generation, it is often very difficult to be certain that no effect at all is present. The preferred basic study design is therefore a two-generation, two-litter study with three dose levels of the test compound, plus a control group. The parental generation should be treated for at least 9 weeks before the second mating, and treatment continued throughout the study. One advantage of deriving the $F_2$ generation from the $F_{1a}$, rather than from the traditional $F_{1b}$ generation, is that an opportunity is available to investigate in detail any effects that may be observed during the mating of the $F_{1a}$ animals. Reproductive performance from mating first litters should be normal, if the animals are not too young at first mating. Normally, not less than 20 males and 20 females should be treated and mated per group. Mating brothers and sisters is not recommended in the last generation. For the earlier generations, larger group sizes should be used to reduce the risk of a concurrent inbreeding bias (Palmer, 1981). All offspring should be reared to weaning, though it is acceptable to reduce the litters to a standard size if desired. At weaning, offspring not involved in producing subsequent generations should be killed and examined macroscopically. In the absence of any gross changes, it is doubtful if there is much to be gained by random measurements of organ weights and histological examination. However, these procedures must be performed if any toxic effect is suspected. It may be advantageous to fix and store the tissues from one male and one female from each litter, at each killing stage, until the study is completed, so that these tissues can be more carefully examined if unexpected toxicity is revealed in the final stages of the study.

#### 4.3.3.3 Choice of species

For economic and temporal reasons, it is usual to perform the above reproduction studies on mice or rats. Ideally, in assessing reproductive toxicity, it should be shown that the species chosen for the reproductive studies metabolize the substances under test by the same routes as man. In practice, this is not always possible (especially with pesticides), but efforts should be made to obtain this information and perform the tests in this way. Where equivocal results are found in rodent studies, tests in other species may be of value. There is no evidence that the results from one particular species or strain extrapolate best to man. Thus, there are no rigid requirements regarding choice of species, but it is very important that adequate control data on reproductive performance should exist for the species used.

#### 4.3.3.4 Doses, route, and duration of treatment

The choice of suitable dose levels is one of the most difficult problems in the design of reproduction tests. The highest dose should induce some signs of general toxicity such as reduced gain in body weight. The lowest dose should be a no-observed-adverse-effect level. Since, usually, only a small percentage of animals are adversely affected, a dose-response relationship is very important in assessing results. Three dose levels are normally required, unless the highest practical dose does not induce any adverse reproductive effect.

The route of administration should be relevant to that in the human exposure. Inhalation exposure for reproductive toxicology has not been widely used and can give rise to misleading results, if undue stress is involved. In such circumstances, alternative routes of administration may be used.

For environmental chemicals such as pesticides, administration throughout the whole period of gestation seems to be the most appropriate, but other treatment regimens are also acceptable.

#### 4.3.3.5 Presentation of results

There is no general agreement on the best statistical method for the analysis of the results of reproductive studies. In the presentation of results, appropriate statistical methods, depending on the distribution of particular endpoint measured, can be used (Snedecor & Cochran, 1967; Sokal & Rohlf, 1969; Hollander & Wolfe, 1973), but it is essential that all of the data for both individual fetuses and litters are presented, so that other methods of assessment can be used if necessary. In all studies, it should be possible to trace the complete outcome of pregnancy in each female.

## 4.4 Transplacental Carcinogenesis

Transplacental carcinogenesis is defined as the appearance of neoplasia in the progeny of females exposed to chemical agents during pregnancy. This phenomenon has been demonstrated in rats, mice, hamsters, rabbits, pigs, dogs, and monkeys with approximately 60 chemicals (Table 11) including representatives of the major classes of chemical carcinogens such as nitroso compounds, polycyclic aromatic hydrocarbons, aminoazo compounds, mycotoxins, and others. While practically all sites of the developing fetuses can be affected by carcinogens administered during pregnancy, the tissues most susceptible to neoplastic responses are those of the nervous system, kidney, and lung. Usually, prenatal susceptibility to carcinogens is greater in the advanced stages of organogenesis; in rodents, for example, it is confined to the last third of the gestational period. With some exceptions specific for certain species or strain (lung adenomas in Swiss mice and some tumours in patas monkeys), tumours do not usually appear before adult life. In at least some tissues, effects of transplacental carcinogens may be enhanced by the application of a carcinogen or promotor to the progeny. In addition, Tomatis (1979) has reported that increased tendency to develop neoplasia may persist without additional exposure, although greatly diminished, in subsequent generations of animals. The same group (Tomatis et al., 1981) has suggested that this transmission may occur via the germ cells, and this is supported by the data of Nomura (1982).

Twenty three compounds and groups of chemicals and 7 industrial processes have been shown to induce carcinogenic effects in human beings (IARC, 1982). However, there is convincing epidemiological evidence of transplacental tumour induction in man for only one compound, i.e., diethylstilboestrol (Herbst et al., 1979a; Rice, 1981).

The following is a summary of the main features of transplacental carcinogenesis in laboratory animals, the research perspectives offered by models under development, and advice on the need for testing compounds in this field.

Table 11. Substances reported to be transplacental carcinogens in animals[a]

| | |
|---|---|
| Polycyclic aromatic hydrocarbons | 7,12-dimethylbenz[a]anthracene<br>benzo[a]pyrene<br>3-methylcholanthrene |
| Aminoazo compounds | 2-fluorenylacetamide<br>2-aminoazotoluene<br>dimethylaminoazobenzene<br>2-toluidine<br>benezidine<br>dichlorobenzidine<br>2-aminotoluene |
| Carbamates | urethane<br>zineb |
| Natural products of plant and animal origin | aflatoxins<br>pyrrolizidine alkaloids<br>cycasin<br>safrol |
| Nitroso compounds | nitrosodimethylamine<br>nitrosodiethylamine<br>nitrosodipropylamine<br>2-hydroxypropylpropylnitrosamine<br>2-oxopropylpropylnitrosamine<br>methylpropylnitrosamine<br>nitrosobis(2-hydroxypropyl) = nitrosamine<br>nitrosodibutylamine<br>4-hydroxybutylbutylnitrosamine<br>nitrosohexamethylenimine<br>nitrosopiperidine<br>dinitrosopiperazine<br>nitrosomethylurea<br>nitrosoethylurea<br>nitrosopropylurea<br>nitrosobutylurea<br>nitrosoethylbiuret<br>nitrosomethylurethane<br>nitrosoethylurethane<br>nitrosobutylurethane |
| Nitroso compounds resulting from interaction of the following precursors | amidopyrine + sodium nitrite<br>diethylamine + sodium nitrite<br>methylurea + sodium nitrite<br>ethylurea + sodium nitrite<br>butylurea + sodium nitrite<br>isopropylurea + sodium nitrite<br>methylbenzylimidazolcarbamate + sodium nitrite<br>citrulline + sodium nitrite<br>propylhexedrine + sodium nitrite |

Table 11 (contd).

| | |
|---|---|
| Other alkylating compounds | azoxymethane<br>azoethane<br>azoxyethane<br>dimethyl sulfate<br>diethyl sulfate<br>1,2-diethylhydrazine<br>1-methyl-2-benzylhydrazine<br>3,3-dimethyl-1-phenyltriazene<br>5-(3,3-dimethyl-1-triazeno) = imidazol-4-carboxamid<br>3,3-diethyl-1-phenyltriazene<br>3,3-diethyl-1-pyridyltriazene<br>3,3 dimethyl-1-pyridyltriazene<br>propane sultone<br>methylmethanesulfonate<br>ethylmethanesulfonate<br>methylazoxymethanol |
| Drugs | diethylstilbestrol<br>carcinolipin<br>cyclophosphamide<br>procarbazine |
| Miscellaneous | tobacco smoke condensate<br>furylfuramide<br>4-oxyphenyllactic acid<br>3-hydroxyxanthine<br>vinyl chloride<br>4-nitroquinoline *N*-oxide |

[a] Data taken from the review by Rice (1981) with additional references for following compounds: nitrosoethylurethane, 3,3-dimethyl-1-pyridyltriazene (Druckrey, 1973), 2-fluorenylacetamide (Armuth & Berenblum, 1977), benzidine (Vesselinovitch et al., 1979), zineb (Kvitnizkaja & Kolesničenko, 1971), pyrrolizidine alkaloids (Schoental & Cavanagh, 1972), dinitrosopiperazine (Börzsönyi et al., 1980), nitrosobutylurea (Maekawa & Odashima, 1975), nitrosobutylurethane (Maekawa et al., 1980), 5-(3,3-dimethyl-1-triazeno)imdazol-4-carboxamide (Zeller, 1980), amidopyrine + sodium nitrite (Alexandrov & Napalkov, 1979), diethylamine + sodium nitrite (Vesselinovitch & Rao, 1974), methylurea + sodium nitrite (Alexandrov, 1973), butylurea + sodium nitrite (Maekawa et al., 1977), isopropylurea + sodium nitrite (Schneider et al., 1977a), methylbenzylimidazolcarbamate + sodium nitrite (Börzönyi et al., 1976), citrulline + sodium nitrite (Ivankovic, 1979), propylhexedrine + sodium nitrite (Schneider et al., 1977b), ethylmethanesulfonate (Schneider et al., 1978), diethylstilboestrol (Rustia & Shubik, 1976; Napalkov & Anisimov, 1979), carcinolipin (Šabad et al., 1973), cyclophosphamide (Roschlau & Justus, 1971), tobacco smoke condensate (Nicolov & Chernozemsky, 1979).

### 4.4.1 Principles and mechanisms of action

#### 4.4.1.1 Comparative sensitivity of the adult and fetal organism to carcinogens

All the transplacental carcinogens that have been studied were already known to be carcinogenic in adult animals. However, the ability of a substance to induce tumours transplacentally can differ in a quantitative way from that observed in weanling or adult animals. For example, it has been established in rats that fetal sensitivity to the action of nitrosoethylurea (NEU) is 20-50 times higher than that of adult animals (Ivankovic & Druckrey, 1968). On the other hand, both fetal and adult rats (Alexandrov, 1969) showed similar sensitivity to nitrosomethylurea (NMU), while sensitivity to the action of nitrosodimethylamine (NDMA) proved to be 6-10 times lower in the fetus than in the adult animal (Alexandrov, 1968). Thus, it appears that the action of chemical carcinogens may be stronger or weaker, after passing through the placenta. A possible explanation is that physico-chemical characteristics of chemical agents affect the rate of transport across the placenta and the biotransformation in the mother and fetus.

Negative results in testing for transplacental carcinogenic effects should be evaluated with caution. It should be kept in mind that the period of development when the rodent embryo is sensitive to carcinogenic stimuli is rather short (10-12 days) and that some compounds require more prolonged application in order to induce tumours.

#### 4.4.1.2 Dependance on the stage of prenatal development

The period of development sensitive to carcinogenesis starts in the advanced stages of organogenesis and lasts until the end of intrauterine life. This has been observed in at least 3 animal species, i.e., the rat (Ivankovic & Druckrey, 1968; Napalkov & Alexandrov, 1968; Alexandrov, 1974), the mouse (Nomura, 1974), and the hamster (Mohr et al., 1975). However, some carcinogens administered to pregnant animals during the early period of embryogenesis, when the placenta has not yet formed, may also induce tumours in the progeny (Spatz & Laqueur, 1967; Nomura, 1974; Börzsönyi et al., 1976; Stavrou et al., 1977).

Generally, transplacental carcinogenesis does not reveal stage specificity for any site in terms of the development and histological appearance of tumours. For example, many chemicals almost exclusively induce tumours of the nervous system and kidney in the rat and of the lung in the mouse, irrespective of the day of exposure.

Susceptibility to transplacental carcinogenesis is influenced by genetic predisposition and appears to be time-specific during pregnancy. Examples of this phenomenon are to be found in rat and mouse studies (Druckrey, 1973; Rice, 1973a; Vesselinovitch, 1973; Alexandrov & Napalkov, 1981). There may be periods of maximal susceptibility that vary from one organ system to another. In the rabbit, for example, the progeny of animals given NEU early in gestation developed brain tumours whereas exposure later in gestation caused only nephroblastoma (Stavrou & Lübbe, 1974; Stavrou et al., 1977).

#### 4.4.1.3 Species and strain specificity

Studies with carcinogenic substances have shown that the type of tumours induced in the progeny differs from species to species. The same agent may induce tumours at different sites, depending on the animal species or strain (Druckery, 1973; Napalkov, 1973; Rice, 1973b; Rice et al., 1979; Ivankovic, 1979). The type of tumours induced transplacentally may or may not necessarily be similar to that induced in adult animals. Among animal species, the most pronounced similarity has been demonstrated in mice (Rice, 1969; Vesselinovitch, 1973; Diwan & Meier, 1974).

Strain dependence has been revealed, even when testing highly organotropic substances. Urethane, which displayed pulmonotropic carcinogenic properties in adult mice, induced transplacentally both lung cancer and tumours at other sites, typical of the strain tested (Vesselinovitch, 1973). The hepatocarcinogen orthoaminoazotoluene, which induced liver tumours transplacentally in certain mouse strains, also often induced tumours of the breast and lung in others (Gelstein, 1961; Golub et al., 1974; Kolesnicenko et al., 1978). Thus organotropism in mice is not only determined by the carcinogenic properties of the compound, but also by strain-specific susceptibility factors. The stage of embryogenesis is also sometimes a determining factor.

In rats, the great majority of substances tested transplacentally, with the exception of symmetrical dialkylnitrosamines, tend to display a pronounced neurotropic carcinogenic effect (Alexandrov, 1976). This great susceptibility of the fetal rat nervous system to transplacental tumour induction by different carcinogenic substances is noteworthy. Kidney tumours also often appeared in rat progeny as a result of transplacental exposure to a number of compounds including 7,12-dimethylbenz(a)anthracene (DMBA), NDMA, *N*-nitrosodiethylamine, NMU, azoxymethane, methylazoxymethanol, 1-methyl-2-benzylhydrazine, procarbazine, and 3,3-dimethyl-1-phenyltriazene (Alexandrov, 1976). It should be noted that all these carcinogenic substances, with the exception of DMBA, are also able to induce kidney tumours in adult animals.

Results of a few studies on rabbits have indicated that the nervous system and kidney of rabbits are sensitive to develop tumours (Güthert et al., 1973; Stavrou & Lubbe, 1974; Beniasvili, 1978). Following transplacental exposure to NEU, monkeys suffered from kidney, soft connective tissue, lung, and nervous system tumours (Rice et al., 1977). Hamsters have been used for assessing the transplacental effects of cigarette condensates and hormones including diethylstilboestrol (Nicolov & Chernozemsky, 1979; Rustia & Shubik, 1976).

#### 4.4.1.4 Mechanisms of organotropism

The mechanism of organotropism displayed by the majority of transplacental carcinogens is poorly understood. Some factors that are believed to contribute to organotropism are:

(a) The predisposition of somatic cells: Little is known about the causes of variation in predisposition and susceptibility among various cell types (Kleihues et al., 1979a);

(b) Metabolic conversion: The extent of metabolic conversion of indirect carcinogens in the whole organism or in the target cells may influence the carcinogenic outcome (Alexandrov & Napalkov, 1981);

(c) Carcinogen-DNA interaction: Cellular DNA is a principle target for carcinogenic chemicals. Studies in transplacental carcinogenesis with ENU, NMU, DMBA, and 3,3-dimethyl-1-phenyltriazene suggest that neoplastic transformation may depend on the degree and persistance of DNA damage in the target tissues (Goth & Rajewsky, 1974; Cooper et al., 1978; Doerjer et al., 1978; Kleihues et al., 1979a; Lihachev et al., 1983). The state of differentiation of target cells at the time of exposure may be important, since the capacity for DNA repair has been shown to change gradually as cells approach the final stages of differentiation (Counis et al., 1977);

(d) Proliferative activity: A relationship has been established between the stage-dependence of the number of lung adenomas induced in fetal mice by exposure to NEU and changes in the number of epithelial cells within the population of cycling cells (Kauffman, 1976). Cells with a high rate of proliferation may be more vulnerable to the action of carcinogenic stimuli as the induced damage is, thus, quickly amplified.

All these factors are closely interrelated since the levels of the enzymes, cell differentiation, and proliferative activity in the target organs are genetically controlled. Altogether, these factors determine both the general sensitivity of the growing organism and the stage specificity of target organs to the insults by carcinogenic agents (Alexandrov & Napalkov, 1981).

#### 4.4.1.5 Metabolism of chemical carcinogens in the maternal organism, the placenta, and the embryo

Tumour development in the offspring is generally determined by the rate of placental transfer, and the concentration of the carcinogen or its active metabolites in the embryonic tissues. It is widely acknowledged that almost all non-ionic organic compounds with a relative molecular mass of less than 600, can cross the placenta (Ginsburg, 1971). There are almost no carcinogenic substances with a relative molecular mass greater than 300 and many are soluble in both lipids and water, which facilitates their transfer across the placenta.

There is no absolute correlation between the accumulation of a given carcinogen in the fetus and the neoplastic response. For example, following administration to pregnant rats, NDMA, a metabolism-dependent carcinogen in adult rats, reaches a high concentration in the fetal tissues, where it remains for almost 24 h (Shendrikova & Alexandrov, 1978). Despite this, however, NDMA is a weak transplacental carcinogen, which suggests that the compound is poorly metabolized by embryonal tissues, probably because of the immaturity of the relevant enzymes. Studies with other carcinogens (polycyclic hydrocarbons and nitroso compounds) have also shown that the concentration of parent chemicals in various embryonic tissues did not correspond with the subsequent incidence of neoplasia in these tissues (Baranova & Alexandrov, 1978).

From experimental data, it appears likely that a transplacental carcinogen acts on the target fetal cells in the following ways (Alexandrov & Napalkov, 1981):

(a) Directly, by reaching the fetus either in its original form or as a spontaneously-formed proximal carcinogen. Examples are nitrosamides, methylazoxymethanol, dimethyl- and diethylsulfate, propane sultone, methylmethanesulphonate. The stability of the initial compounds or their proximal derivatives is the limiting factor. Methylnitrosourethane (MNU) when given to pregnant rats failed to induce carcinogenic effects in the progeny, because of its rapid degradation in the mother. However, the carcinogenic effect was readily induced following intra-amniotic administration and direct injection into fetal rats (Alexandrov, 1972; Napalkov, 1973);

(b) Indirectly, by generating proximal carcinogens in target fetal cells through metabolic activation. Examples are dialkylnitrosamines, 1,2-dialkylhydrazines, azo- and azoxy-alkanes, and procarbazine. In this case, the metabolic capacity of the target cells is a limiting factor. In particular, NDMA, when administered to pregnant rats, induced no teratogenic effects and only a weak transplacental carcinogenic effect. These findings were ascribed to the incomplete metabolic development of the rat fetuses (Alexandrov, 1968; Napalkov, 1973). When the active metabolites of enzyme-dependent carcinogens are short-lived, the enzymatic capability of the target fetal cells acquires primary importance;

(c) Indirectly, following maternal metabolism. A stable proximal carcinogen may be formed and pass through the placenta. Examples are cyclophosphamide (Hales, 1982), and 3,3-dimethyl-1-phenytriazine (Kleihues, 1979b), which are metabolized in the maternal liver, and cycasin, which is metabolized by maternal intestinal flora (Laqueur & Spatz, 1973);

(d) Indirectly, by the production of proximal and ultimate carcinogenic metabolites in the placenta. This mode of action is not well documented though polycyclic hydrocarbons are known to undergo metabolic activation in the placenta (Welch et al., 1969; Pelkonen et al., 1972; Sehgal & Hutton, 1977), and may belong to this class.

Transplacental carcinogenesis can also occur as a result of the formation of nitroso compounds from their precursors in the stomach of pregnant females (Table 11). The carcinogenic action on the fetus occurs via (c) and (a), in the case of ethylurea and nitrite administration, and according to types (c) and (b), in the case of amidopyrine and nitrite administration.

### 4.4.2 Relationship between teratogenesis and carcinogenesis

There are a number of compounds that have both carcinogenic and teratogenic properties (Neubert, 1980b). This is not surprising when considering electrophilic substances such as alkylating agents, which react with many cell components. However, teratogenic activity has not been observed for every carcinogen, nor would this be expected. Though the possibility of common steps in teratogenesis and carcinogenesis exists, there are probably specific mechanisms pertinent to only one or other of these phenomena. In studies in which rats were tested with a combination of NMU and NEU, it was established that the development of malformations of the hypoplastic type (microcephaly) did not prevent the appearance of brain tumours, and that the phenomena of teratogenesis and carcinogenesis could coexist, but were apparently independent (Alexandrov & Napalkov, 1976).

In most cases, since malformations and tumours are induced in different organs, there is no reason to assume that the two processes are related. In clinical/epidemiological observations (Miller, 1977), diethylstilboestrol is the only compound shown to have caused malformations (adenosis), and malignant tumours (clear cell adenocarcinomas) in the same organs, the cervix and vagina. The sensitive period for the induction of these carcinogenic and teratogenic effects was the same (Herbst et al., 1979b). The immature opossum is the only animal model developed to date that has provided clear-cut indications that malformations can be produced together with embryonal tumours in the same organs (Jurgelski et al., 1976).

### 4.4.3 General principles of transplacental carcinogenicity tests

A compound found to be carcinogenic in adult carcinogenicity studies does not usually need testing for transplacental carcinogenicity. However, it may be worth investigating the relative adult versus fetal sensitivity for chemicals to which many pregnant women have been, or are, unavoidably exposed. As a primary task, compounds that are suspected of being human carcinogens (IARC, 1982), should be tested for transplacental carcinogenicity.

The general guidelines for conducting transplacental carcinogenicity studies do not differ considerably from those adopted for adult animal studies (IARC, 1980). Some substances may prove inactive in conventional test systems. This could be because the period of development during which the rodent embryo is sensitive to carcinogenic stimuli is rather short (during last 10-12 days of pregnancy) and these compounds may require prolonged application to induce tumours. Therefore, care should be taken in extrapolating negative results from animal studies to man, and appropriate models with non-human primates or other suitable mammalian species should be developed. Variables that should be taken into account include: species and strain, stage of pregnancy, dose and route of administration, period of observation, registration of biological variables (e.g., body weight) and statistical evaluation of the results. The following experimental conditions are peculiar to transplacental studies.

#### 4.4.3.1 Species

It is advisable to use at least two laboratory species, preferably mice and rats. The sensitivity of fetal rats to direct and indirect carcinogens varies and is manifested with a rather peculiar organ specificity that is not typical of adult animals. On the other hand, the sensitivity of fetal mice to the transplacental action of carcinogens does not differ significantly from the sensitivity of adult mice, and neoplasms usually appear at sites typical for spontaneous tumours.

In some studies, other species, including hamsters, have been used. For economic reasons, non-human primates should be reserved for studies on the mechanisms of prenatal carcinogenesis related to human beings.

#### 4.4.3.2 Stages of pregnancy

The period of optimum susceptibility during pregnancy of a test species should be chosen as the duration of treatment with the test agent. The following two experimental designs could be recommended for mice, hamsters, and rats: (a) single exposure, 1-5 days before parturition; and (b) multiple exposures, daily from day 11 to the end of pregnancy (Alexandrov & Napalkov, 1981). In monkeys (*Erythrocebus patas*), the period between days 30-50 of pregnancy may be selected, since this period has been shown to be quite effective in transplacental studies (Rice et al., 1977).

#### 4.4.3.3 Dose and route of administration

To select an appropriate route, toxicokinetic peculiarities should be given particular consideration. For example, substances that are slowly absorbed from the site of administration should be tested by means of a course of treatment. However, for practical purposes, it is advisable to use two different routes, namely intravenous and oral.

Doses should be selected from pilot tests in which mortality, body weight gain, and other pathological alterations in mothers and offspring, have been evaluated. Administration of the maximum tolerable dose may provide early and pronounced carcinogenic effects, while a series of lower doses will help to reveal a "dose-effect" relationship, which is important for extrapolating and evaluating the carcinogenic risk for human beings.

The number of pregnant females in each group should be large enough to provide for not less than 50 offspring per sex. The offspring of treated and control mothers should be cross-fostered to ascertain that the carcinogenic effect of a chemical is transplacental, unless postnatal transfer from mother to offspring can be excluded.

#### 4.4.3.4 Evaluation of results

The progeny should be followed up for the entire life-span of the species under consideration, neoplastic changes being analysed by histological examination of the affected organs and tissues, at the end of the study. A reliable source for classifying the tumours has been provided by IARC (Turusov, 1973, 1976, 1979, 1982). Attention should be paid to other toxic manifestations including dystrophy, necrosis, atrophy, malformations, dishormonal status, etc. Methods for the statistical evaluation of results have been described (IARC, 1980).

### 4.4.4 Methods with potential for the future

#### 4.4.4.1 Transplacental host-mediated cell culture

This system offers a means for the rapid screening of compounds, including those requiring metabolic activation, for possible transplacental carcinogenicity. In cells subcultured from embryonal tissues, following administration of chemicals to animals during pregnancy, signs of morphological transformation may be detected several weeks after *in vitro* growth (Quarles, 1981). In another model, the activity of a chemical may be determined according to the marked induction of mutants resistant to 8-azaguanine in a culture of embryo cells derived from pregnant animals treated with the test compound (Endo et al., 1980).

#### 4.4.4.2 Pre- and postnatal exposure to carcinogens and promoting factors

A few studies have shown an increased carcinogenic effect when an initial prenatal exposure to a carcinogen was followed by postnatal exposure to either a carcinogen (Lichachev, 1971) or a promoting agent (Goerttler & Loehrke, 1976), or by hormonal imbalance (Alexandrov & Anisimov, 1976). This approach could be useful for determining the carcinogenic potential of chemicals with marginal effects in adult animals (Napalkov, 1973).

4.4.4.3 Intraamniotic and intrafetal injection technique

This procedure distinguishes between the direct effects of a test compound on the fetus and the effects induced following maternal treatment. The high susceptibility of rodent fetal cells to some of the carcinogens administered directly into the fetus suggests that intraamniotic or intrafetal injections might find useful applications in detecting potentially hazardous chemicals (Alexandrov & Napalkov, 1981; Rossi et al., 1983).

# 5. *IN VITRO* DEVELOPMENTAL AND NON-MAMMALIAN ANIMAL SYSTEMS: CURRENT AND FUTURE APPLICATIONS

Various *in vitro* developmental systems (cell, organ, and whole embryo culture) have been used to investigate the morphological and biochemical basis for normal and abnormal development. Such systems are extremely useful for this sort of basic and applied research. The current demands on whole animal testing systems may prevent testing of all the rapidly increasing number of chemical agents being introduced into the environment.

Short-term tests using various *in vitro* and *in ovo* systems might offer a future means of selecting chemical agents for subsequent teratology testing in animals. Short-term *in vitro* methods and their applicability have been reviewed by Rajan (1974), Kochhar (1975a), Saxén & Saxén (1975), Ebert & Marois, ed. (1976), Wilson (1978a, b), Barrach & Neubert (1980), Neubert (1980a), Neubert & Merker, ed. (1981), Kimmel et al. (1982), Neubert (1982), Neubert (1983), and Shepard et al. (1983).

## 5.1 Scope of In Vitro Developmental Systems

These studies are carried out using a variety of biological systems (Table 13), capable of reflecting normal developmental processes.

It is evident that, within the last decade, several culture techniques, especially those using mammalian tissues, have been successfully applied to the elucidation of basic mechanisms occurring at the biochemical and cellular levels during embryonic development, and to a closer analysis of the modes of teratogenic action. There is no doubt that *in vitro* methods have greatly broadened the possibilities in this field of research. *In vitro* systems can be considered from three points of view (Neubert, 1981; Kimmel et al., 1982; Neubert, 1982): (a) as foods for the elucidation of mechanisms relevant to normal and abnormal development; (b) as tools for obtaining information on dose responses and specific organ toxicity; (c) as foods for the selection of chemicals for possible future developmental toxicity testing. *In vitro* developmental systems are attractive for toxicological studies as many are relatively inexpensive, and they are easier to perform and less time-consuming than whole-animal studies. However, a number of problems need to be solved before using Short-Term Selection Tests (STST) routinely. *In vitro* developmental systems, applicable to studies or problems concerning basic developmental biology, must be able to mimic certain processes characteristic of prenatal or perinatal development.

## 5.2 Essential and Desirable Features of Short-Term Selection Tests

Essential and desirable features of STST, summarized in Table 12, have been proposed by several investigators (Wilson, 1977; Kimmel et al., 1982; Neubert, 1982; Shepard et al., 1983).

The injudicious use of in vitro test data could be even more dangerous than extrapolation from routine in vivo tests. Excessive false positives could lead to an undesirable situation in which in vivo test systems in use, would be overburdened. Some false negatives are bound to occur, but they must be small in number, otherwise there is little purpose in the STST.

A simpler system is preferable to a whole organism, only if the underlying toxic mechanism is largely understood, occurs universally, and can be completely mimicked. In the short-term tests used in mutagenicity studies, these prerequisites seem to have been fulfilled to some extent but, even here, no single test system has been found to be fully adequate. The situation in prenatal toxicity is more complex than in mutagenicity, since numerous mechanisms are known to lead to abnormal development. Thus, no one test system is likely to identify all the abnormal reactions that may occur.

The culture technique, if chosen, will largely depend on the problem to be solved. If, for example, cell interactions and their disturbance by certain agents are to be studied, cell cultures or techniques using cell suspensions may be the method of choice. Specific embryonic differentiation processes (palate closure, limb development, kidney development) may be best studied with organ culture techniques,

Table 12. Features of a short-term selection test (STST)

| | |
|---|---|
| Essential | Results must be predictive of in vivo effects<br>Few false positives<br>Very few false negatives<br>Inexpensive and readily-available biological unit<br>Easily quantificated endpoint<br>Reproducibility of results between laboratories |
| Desirable | Incorporating as many developmental processes as possible by using a series or battery of tests<br>Ability to test water-soluble and water-insoluble chemicalsand gaseous agents<br>Ability to determine dose-response relationships<br>Ability to incorporate biotransforming systems, especially hepatic monooxygenase systems, from different species including man |

whereas processes of cell migration over long distances within the embryo may be best studied in whole embryo cultures. In many instances, the results obtained are only valid within the limits of the model and for the species used.

In short-term tests, it is difficult or impossible to establish the relationship between embryo/fetal toxicity and maternal toxicity, which is essential for determining whether the effects are selective or not. In addition, many compounds are metabolically activated to electrophilic substances that react with cell constituents and thereby cause toxicity. This activation may occur in the embryo/fetus or the mother, or in both. The role of enzyme induction in the mother and the conceptus is another important issue. The addition of metabolizing enzyme systems from different species may make it possible for investigators to obtain information on inter-species differences (Fantel et al., 1979; Neubert, 1982; Shepard et al., 1983). This method might be especially valuable in extrapolating from experimental animals to human beings, even though this approach will not fully reproduce metabolism *in vivo*.

The influence of the mother on the toxic effects in the fetus is difficult to reproduce in an *in vitro* system. This is also true of chick embryos *in ovo*, which are used for the assessment of the embryotoxic potential of chemicals. The maternal factor is highly relevant if little is known of the toxicokinetics of a given chemical - as is the case with many chemicals in the environment.

### 5.3 Validation of Short-Term Selection Tests

To be accepted as part of a routine testing process, STSTs will have to be validated for their ability to predict the teratogenic potential of an agent. For the purpose of validation, necessary criteria will have to be developed, the number and type of chemicals (representative of diverse structures and biological activities) required for testing will have to be decided, and an acceptable percentage of false positives and false negatives will need to be agreed upon. To carry out validation in a controlled fashion and to facilitate interlaboratory comparisons, a list of chemicals to be used should be developed jointly by scientists experienced in teratology, toxicokinetics, and biochemistry. An attempt to choose agents that are teratogenic or non-teratogenic has been undertaken by Smith et al. (in press).

Final validation of tests to be used must be based on the results of the *in vitro* tests of known human teratogens. Up to the present, no STSTs have been fully validated and no recommendations are made in this document as to which batteries of STSTs are likely to emerge for possible use in the future. The STSTs are not in any way intended to replace animal tests, but merely to supplement them so that they can be made more efficient and productive.

## 5.4 Available Developmental Systems

Some developmental systems that are in use at present for basic mechanism studies, or proposed as STSTs (Table 13) are discussed in section 5.4.1. None of these developmental systems involves the chorioallantoic placenta or an intact maternal metabolic system. In some cases, a mono-oxygenase or other type of bioactivating system may be added. A summary of many of these developmental systems has been published by Neubert (1982).

### 5.4.1 Whole-embryo culture (warm-blooded animals)

There are three types of cultures that have been used extensively in various laboratories:

(a) culture of mammalian preimplantation stages;

(b) culture of mammalian postimplantation embryos; and

(c) culture of non-mammalian (avian) embryos.

Though not a culture method, the evaluation of the chick embryo *in ovo* will also be discussed.

#### 5.4.1.1 Ovum maturation and preimplantation stages

*In vitro* maturation of the ovum of different mammalian species (especially rodents) has been intensively studied (Edwards, 1980; Edwards & Purdy, 1982). With this system it is possible to investigate the mechanism of action of various chemicals on chromosomal disjunction, ovum maturation, and activation. It is possible to use *in vitro* fertilization of human ova not only as a method of treating human infertility, but also to obtain a better understanding of the basic mechanism of human oogenesis (Edwards, 1980; Kurilo et al., 1982, 1983).

Culture of cleaving mammalian ova is being used to study the mechanism of embryotoxic action of some chemicals, especially those that are expected to influence proliferation and induce chromosomal aberrations (Dyban et al., 1976, 1977a,b; Spielmann et al., 1981; Matsumoto & Spindle, 1982).

Hsu (1979, 1980, 1981) published results of a system in which it is possible to study mammalian development *in vitro* from the preimplantation phase to the late embryonic stages.

Table 13. Developmental systems

| System | Period of development covered | Developmental process studied and endpoint |
|---|---|---|
| I. Whole-embryo culture | | |
| Mammalian embryos (including human) | preimplantation | fertilization, cleavage, and blastocyst formation |
| Rodent embryos | post-implantation organogenesis | organogenesis over 2 (or 3) days |
| Chick embryo culture | organogenesis | organogenesis |
| Chick embryo *in ovo* | entire | whole development |
| Amphibian embryos | entire | whole development |
| Zebra fish | entire | whole development |
| II. Organ cultures | | |
| Limb buds (avian, rodents) | late organogenesis | morphogenesis cartilage formation muscle formation |
| Palatal shelves | organogenesis | epithelial fusion and cell death, palate closure |
| Tooth bud | organogenesis | dental development, histogenesis of tooth buds |
| Lens | organogenesis | lens differentiation, histogenesis, and protein production |
| Pancreas | organogenesis | acinar development, histogenesis, biochemical development |
| Sex organs | late organogenesis | gonadal and organ development, germ cell maturation, accessory sex gland, histogenesis |
| Kidney | late organogenesis | nephrogenesis, histogenesis |
| Thyroid | late organogenesis | thyroid, histogenesis, and functional development |

Table 13 (contd).

| | | |
|---|---|---|
| III. Tissue culture | | |
| Chick neural crest | organogenesis | migration and pigmentation, melanin formation or acethylcholine transferase activity |
| Chick limb bud mesenchyme | organogenesis | growth and chondrogenesis |
| Lung micromass culture | organogenesis | pattern formation, cell recognition, and adhesion |
| Embryonic heart | organogenesis | histogenesis and functions |
| Skeletal muscle | organogenesis | myogenesis, cell fusion, and histogenesis |
| Teratocarcinoma | organogenesis | histogenesis |
| Mouse tumour cells | none | cell attachment |
| Human embryonic cell culture | organogenesis | growth of patatal mesenchymal cells |
| IV. Invertebrates | | |
| *Hydra attenuae* | adult and embryonic | aggregation and movement regeneration of damaged and disassociated adults |
| *Drosophila melanogaster* | entire | myogenesis, nerve attachment |
| *Planaria* | regeneration of adult | neurogenesis, eye development |
| Sea urchins | cleavage | cell replications and contacts |
| *Dictyostelium* | entire | aggregation, differentiation |
| V. Other approaches | | |
| Amphibian limb adult regeneration | differentiation | myogenesis, neurogenesis, and chondrogenesis |
| Virus | unknown | (viral replication) |
| Lipophilic or electrophilic chemical property | unknown | (cell membrane penetration, toxic potential) |

However, the success rate of this model has not yet exceeded 10%. In general, preimplantation embryos cannot be cultured beyond stages corresponding to implantation or early postimplantation.

It is now possible to culture mammalian embryos from the one- or two-cell stage to the blastocyst stage. Most of the work has been performed with the preimplantation stages of mice (McLaren & Biggers, 1958; Brinster, 1963; Runner, 1965; Biggers et al., 1971; Whitten, 1971; Whittingham, 1971; Eibs & Spielmann, 1977; Speilmann & Eibs, 1977), but cultivation of preimplanted rat, rabbit, and human embryos has also been carried out successfully (Brachet, 1913; Chang, 1949; Daniel, 1965; Daniel, Jr, 1968; Mauer et al., 1968; Onuma et al., 1968; Edwards et al., 1969; Brinster, 1970; Steptoe & Edwards, 1978; Edwards & Purdy, 1982). A chemically-defined, serum-free, culture medium is generally used for this purpose.

Biophysical and biochemical techniques have been used in addition to morphological and biochemical methods to analyse the normal and abnormal development of preimplantation stages. The measuring of membrane potentials has been used as an indication of functional stage in the eggs of sea urchins and mammals (Crose et al., 1973; Leonov et al., 1972, 1975; Persianinov et al., 1973).

Most investigators agree that the preimplantation period is not sensitive to the induction of gross structural abnormalities (Austin, 1973). Preimplantation embryos, therefore, have not been used much in teratology. However, abnormal development associated with early or delayed mortality can be induced before implantation (cf. Snow, 1973, 1975; Goldstein et al., 1975; Spielmann et al., 1981; Pedersen, 1981).

Many drugs may reach the preimplantation embryo via the tubal or uterine fluids, and agents, such as nicotine, may even accumulate within the blastocyst (Fabro, 1973; Sieber & Fabro, 1974). Lutwak-Mann (1973), has suggested the use of "flat mounts" of rabbit blastocysts to detect abnormalities induced by embryotoxic agents, but this technique has not gained acceptance.

#### 5.4.1.2 Postimplantation mammalian embryos

Developed by New and co-workers (New, 1966a,b, 1976, 1978; New et al., 1976a,b), the culture of whole rodent embryos *in vitro* is now an established procedure in many laboratories. Mouse or rat embryos are cultured with their embryonic membranes intact by the rotating bottle technique (New et al., 1973; Cockroft & Coppola, 1977), which is generally preferred to more sophisticated experimental procedures. Rat embryos (8.5 - 10.5-day-old), can be cultured over a 24-h or even a 48-h period and embryonic stages corresponding to about

35-somites may be reached. Up to the 30-somite stage, the development proceeds at roughly the same rate in vitro as in vivo. Abnormal development may occur in culture, if conditions are inadequate.

Some studies have been conducted on mice (Clarkson et al., 1969; Sadler, 1979a,b; Davis et al., 1981) and on hamster embryos (Givelber & Dipaolo, 1968). Rat embryos have been traditionally cultured in a medium containing rat serum, but some investigators have successfully grown them in human serum (Shepard et al., 1969; Chatot et al, 1980; Klein et al., 1980, 1981; Herken & Anschütz, 1981), dialysed serum (Clarkson et al., 1969; Gunberg, 1976), and in a chemically-defined serum-free medium (Klee-Trieschmann & Neubert, 1981). In several studies, the direct embryotoxic potential of teratogens for the developing embryo was elucidated following their addition to the culture medium (for bibliography see Neubert, 1982). Popov et al. (1981) and Fantel (1982) used a liver microsomal system added to the culture to activate cyclophosphamide. Dyban as well as Klein and his co-workers studied the effects on embryos in a culture serum containing a variety of compounds (e.g., cyclophosphamide), which had been obtained from animals treated in vivo or from patients (Dyban, 1977; Dyban et al., 1979; Klein et al., 1980, 1981). Only gross morphological evaluations were performed in most of the studies. A morphological scoring system (Brown et al., 1980) may be useful for evaluation, but, for more detailed analysis, histological examination is essential (Herken & Anschütz, 1981). A technique of culturing whole embryos in which it is possible to the record the embryonic heart beat has been developed (Robkin et al., 1972). An attempt has also been made to use a sequence of whole-embryo cultures with subsequent organ culturing of, for example, limb buds (Kochhar, 1976). The applicability of the whole-embryo technique as a routine method is limited, because it is expensive, too sensitive to disturbances, often of unknown origin, and quite prone to abnormal development, even under normal conditions. Furthermore, a maximum culture period of 48 h is often too short compared with the entire period of organogenesis. The method is especially useful for studying certain aspects of developmental biology, such as the nutrient requirements of embryos during organogenesis, or for performing biochemical analyses or studies with radioactively-labelled precursors (Shepard et al., 1970).

#### 5.4.1.3 Chick embryo in culture

Explantation of the early chick embryo is technically more difficult than culturing embryonic mammals at the preimplantation stages. The problems involved, however, have mostly been solved in the technique of New (1955; 1966a,b). It consists of supporting the explanted blastoderm on a piece of vitelline membrane stretched across a glass ring. The ring is placed on a watch glass serving as a reservoir for nutrient medium - thin albumen, obtained perhaps from the same donor egg. The watch glass is kept in a covered Petri dish, which forms a moist chamber. Primitive streak blastoderms explanted by this technique develop at a normal rate for approximately 48 h, until after the 20-somite stage. Agents can be tested by direct addition to the medium, and sera from individuals exposed to the agent can be added to the culture. Embryos examined for toxic effects are examined for changes in size and gross morphology, histology, and biochemical variables such as DNA and protein content, glucose consumption and lactate production, cellular damage, etc. (New, 1976). This method is inexpensive and can be used routinely with standard laboratory equipment. Large numbers of embryos can be processed in a short time.

Since the embryos can only be maintained for a relatively short period of time, the usefulness of this technique is limited to the early developmental stages. Effects caused by substances acting mainly or entirely at later developmental stages cannot be detected by this procedure.

#### 5.4.1.4 Chick embryo in ova

Chemicals have frequently been tested in chick embryos, at all stages of development, by administration into fertile eggs. A chemical, in solution or suspension, is usually deposited on the air-sac membrane or injected into the yolk and the chicks examined before or after hatching. This method has often failed to supply reliable results as it has been difficult to standardize the blind injection technique. Moreover, it is doubtful whether the form and concentration of a chemical, when it reaches the embryo, is known. A standard window technique for delivering the chemical to the chick embryo has been developed for embryotoxicity and teratogenicity studies in which better control of experimental conditions is possible (Jelinek et al., 1976; Jelinek, 1979; Jelinek & Peterka, 1981). The test substance is administered in a single application to the subgerminal portion of the yolk of the embryo on day 2, and intra-amniotically on days 3 or 4. The number of dead, malformed, and growth-retarded embryos is counted on the eighth day of incubation, when the study is terminated. The method is inexpensive and requires a moderate degree of skill. The effect of a large number of variables can be assessed and the amount of the test chemical needed is small. With this test it is possible to determine dose-response and stage-response relationships and the affinity of a substance for particular organ systems. The capacity of the system for the metabolic activation of xenobiotics is ill-defined. Testing of compounds that are insoluble or soluble in toxic solvents is difficult and false-positives are common with surface-active compounds. Though many compounds have so far been tested in chick ova, the predictive value of these tests has not yet been established.

### 5.4.2 Organ cultures

The term organ culture should be used when a whole-organ anlagen, or its representative part (e.g., a lobe of a lung or liver), is kept in culture and growth, particularly organ-specific differentiation, is observed. Two approaches have been used:

(a) the explant, is kept on a filter or other support, and differentiates at the interface of the culture medium and the gas phase (Trowell, 1961); and

(b) the explant is submerged in the culture medium, and shaking or rotation is used to guarantee gas exchange and diffusion.

Both of these techniques show a number of advantages and certain disadvantages depending on the embryonic organ or organ anlage used. The successful use of organ culture systems in developmental biology and toxicology has recently been reviewed (Neubert, 1982). Serum-containing medium has been employed in the majority of cases, but successful attempts have been made to culture certain tissues in chemically-defined media.

The technique described by Trowell (1961) has been used in the culture of a variety of tissues and organs from mammalian or avian embryos or fetuses. It is comparatively easy to perform and 100-200 explants can be prepared by one person in one day. A modification of the method, the trans-filter technique, is used for induction studies (Grobstein, 1956; Saxén et al., 1968; Wartiovaara et al., 1974; Saxén & Lehtonen, 1978).

#### 5.4.2.1 Organ culture of limb buds

The Trowell technique is used for the culture of limb buds from rat or mouse embryos (Shepard & Bass, 1970; Kochhar, 1970; Aydelotte & Kochhar, 1972) but it may also be used for limb buds from embryos of other species, e.g., rabbit, chick, or ferret (Lessmöllmann et al., 1975; Beck & Gulamhusein,

1980a). Growth of limb buds in culture, is retarded compared with in vivo development, but morphological differentiation of the cartilaginous bone anlagen and of muscle can be observed. With any of these techniques, the extent of the morphogenetic differentiation of the cartilaginous bone anlagen depends largely on the stage of development at which the cultures are initiated. In earlier studies, serum-containing medium was used, but more recently a chemically-defined medium has been preferred (Lessmöllmann et al., 1975, 1976).

The submerged culture system has also been successfully used for the study of limb bud differentiation in vitro (Neubert & Barrach, 1977b; Blankenburg et al., 1981), and it shows many advantages over the Trowell technique. Dissected limb buds can be stored at low temperatures for several weeks (Neubert & Bluth, 1981a) and some studies may be facilitated by the use of such an organ bank. This organ culture technique is one of the best and most extensively studied. Normal development and differentiation, predominantly of the cartilaginous bone anlagen, have been studied and a variety of morphological (e.g., Merker, 1975; Merker et al., 1978b; Neubert et al., 1974a, 1976) and biochemical (e.g., Rautenberg & Neubert, 1975; Neubert & Rautenberg, 1976; Barrach et al., 1975, 1980, 1981; Blankenburg et al., 1980, 1981, Dusemund & Barrach, 1981) variables have been evaluated. Although the amount of protein increases within the explants, there is little or no increase in the total DNA (Neubert et al., 1976).

It has been possible to induce abnormal development in vitro by adding a variety of teratogens to the culture medium (Kochhar, 1970, 1975b; Aydelotte & Kochhar, 1972; Neubert et al., 1974b, 1976, 1977a; Barrach et al., 1978; Merker et al., 1978a; Welsch et al., 1978; Merker & Günther, 1979; Beck & Gulamhusein, 1980b; Bochert et al., 1981; Neubert & Bluth, 1981b; Stahlmann et al., 1981, 1983).

It has also been possible to quantify the extent of differentiation achieved in culture and to establish dose-response relationships for abnormal development using the organ culture system. Biochemical variables, such as levels of DNA, RNA, protein, collagen, etc. can be measured (Neubert et al., 1974a); or a score system may be used for morphogenetic differentiation (Neubert et al., 1977a; 1978b). Image analysis (Kwasigroch et al., 1981) can also be used to quantify abnormal development.

#### 5.4.2.2 Organ culture of the pancreas

Organ culture has been used by Rutter and his colleagues (Pictet & Rutter, 1972; Rutter et al., 1975) to study the development of the embryonic rat pancreas. The information gained using this system has provided the most extensive biochemical background for any prenatally developing mammalian tissue investigated so far. However, the pancreas is not considered a major target for embryo- or fetotoxic agents.

### 5.4.2.3 Organ culture of palatal shelves

Growth and differentiation of the palatal shelves has also been achieved in organ culture. This system has been extensively used to study cleft palate-inducing agents (Lahti & Saxén, 1967, 1972; Saxén, 1973; Fairbanks & Kollar, 1974; Pratt et al., 1980; Brinkley, 1980; Pratt, 1983).

### 5.4.2.4 Organ culture of tooth anlagen

Normal and abnormal development of tooth anlagen has been studied, both morphologically and biochemically, using the organ culture technique. Important information on connective tissue development and on the induction of abnormalities has been obtained (Ruch & Karcher-Djuricic, 1971; Kollar, 1973; Galbraith & Kollar, 1974; Koch, 1974; Hetem et al., 1975; Kerley & Kollar, 1978; Thesleff & Pratt, 1980).

### 5.4.2.5 Organ culture of the embryonic lens

Lens development can be followed using human embryonic material. The induction of abnormal development by rubella virus can be mimicked in vitro. Cataract formation was observed by Karkinen-Jääskeläinen et al. (1975).

### 5.4.2.6. Organ culture of the embryonic kidney

Organ culture techniques have been developed for the study of explanted mouse or human embryonic kidney (Saxén, 1965; Saxén et al., 1968; Crocker & Vernier, 1970; Crocker, 1973; Saxén & Lehtonen, 1978; Saxén & Ekblom, 1981). This system may prove useful for investigating the normal mechanisms of renal development and also testing suspected nephrotoxic agents. The expense and time involved are both fairly high, since the endpoints require histological analysis.

### 5.4.2.7 Organ culture of embryonic gonads and accessory duct systems

Organ culture of embryonic gonads together with assessory ducts has contributed to the understanding of how hormones and some hormone inhibitors modify sexual development (Martinovitch, 1938; Jost & Bergerard, 1949; Price & Ortiz, 1965; Josso, 1974; Lasnitzki & Mizuno, 1981). Both mammalian and avian embryos have been used. These techniques could be used to investigate new chemicals that might have specific effects on the genital system. The method is moderately expensive and time-consuming.

5.4.2.8 Organ culture of thyroid tissue

Tissue from the thyroid glands or their embryonic primordia from chick, rodents, and human beings may be explanted into organ cultures, which may then be exposed to hormones and various xenobiotics. The effects can be studied biochemically or histochemically (Shepard, 1965, 1967, 1974). Appearance of colloid within thyroid follicles, histoautoradiography of incorporated radioiodine, or biochemical analysis of various labelled organic compounds are used for evaluation. The expense and time required are moderate. This test system would be of use in investigating very specific questions about the effects of new chemicals on gland maturation and function.

5.4.2.9 Other organ culture systems

The use of organ culture is not restricted to the examples provided in the preceeding paragraphs and other organ anlagen have been cultured. Examples include the use of bone from rat or mouse fetuses (to demonstrate the pathological developments induced by substances such as glucocorticoids or tetracycline) (Fell & Weiss, 1965; Saxén, 1966; Saxén & Kaitila, 1972), digits (Rajan, 1969, 1974; Rajan et al., 1980), lung anlagen (Riso & Zimmermann, 1981), intestine (Silano et al., 1981), and liver (Räihä & Schwartz, 1973).

5.4.3 Culture of non-mammalian or non-avian embryos

Embryos of amphibia, lurchae, or fish have been extensively used in research (New, 1966b), but only a few of these systems have been suggested as models for the evaluation of embryotoxic risks. Some of these animal models are listed below, though these species are much less favourable for the routine testing of potential embryotoxic agents, as their response to such agents has not been properly investigated, so far.

5.4.3.1 Studies on the development of fish

Several species of fish have been studied embryologically and at least two species, Oryzias and zebra fish, have been used for studies on abnormal development (Smithberg, 1962; Schreiweis & Murray, 1976; Leung & Bulkley, 1979). Streisinger (1975) proposed using zebra fish for the study of teratogens. By fertilizing eggs with genetically-inactive sperm and blocking their first mitotic division, homozygous diploid embryos can be obtained, some of which develop into adult forms. Clones of the fish can be established, which may be useful in dose-response analysis. The raising and study of the wild form of zebra fish might prove to be inexpensive and not too time-consuming. So far, not much information on teratogenicity has been obtained from these studies, but they may be valuable for the evaluation of the effects of environmental chemicals on wild life.

#### 5.4.3.2 Studies on the development of amphibia, lurchae, sea-urchins, and other invertebrates

None of these systems has been adequately analysed for responsiveness to toxic substances. The species observed in developmental studies include: amphibia (Schultz et al., 1982), *Drosophila* (Demerec, 1950), sea urchins (Lallier, 1965) and worms (Deppe et al., 1978). Sea urchin eggs have been the subject of reproduction studies, because synchronically developing embryos can be obtained in large numbers (Harvey, 1956; Costello et al., 1957; Mateyko, 1967) and experimental conditions (fertilization and incubation) are simple (Tyler & Tyler, 1966; Hinegarduer, 1967; Reverby, 1971; Hörstadium, 1973). It is possible to study embryotoxic and teratogenic effects (Hagström & Lönning, 1973; Leonov, 1979) and many chemical substances can easily penetrate the external coats of eggs and embryos.

*Hydra attenuae* has been recommended as a model for developmental toxicity testing but, in this case, it is not the development that is studied. *Hydra attenuata* are grown in trays and are fed *Artemia nauplii* (Johnson, 1980; Johnson et al., 1982). Two endpoints can be measured after addition of a chemical agent to the liquid medium. One endpoint, representing the adult toxic dose, is an irreversible morphological alteration called the "tulip" stage. With the second, artificial "embryos" are formed by compacting dissociated adult cells (Gierer et al., 1972) and dissolution of the aggregates is the endpoint of the test. The expense is small and little time is required. If the system can be validated, it might prove useful in evaluating large numbers of substances.

### 5.4.4 Tissue culture systems

The use of tissue culture systems in developmental toxicology is limited, but primary cultures from various embryonic tissues have been extensively used in developmental studies including the chick neural crest (Greenberg, 1982), heart mesenchymal cells, and skeletal muscle cells (Holtzer et al., 1958). Cell lines can be used in developmental toxicology. They may be employed in testing for the general cytotoxicity of chemical. However, it must be remembered that some cells may change their characteristics in culture. Pratt et al. (1980) have used an established cell line from the human embryonic palatal mesenchyme (HEPM) to aid in understanding the biochemical basis for the way in which glucocorticoids inhibit palatal mesenchymal cell growth and cause cleft palate in the rodent. Furthermore, Pratt et al. (1982) have suggested that teratogen-induced growth inhibition in these HEPM cells might be used as part of a battery of assays to screen for potential environmental teratogens.

It seems possible that, in some instances, primary cell cultures of embryonic or fetal cells - including those from human embryos or fetuses - may be used for studies on the drug-metabolizing capacity of cells during prenatal, and especially perinatal, development (Nau et al., 1977; Egger et al., 1978; Liddiard et al., 1978; Merker et al., 1978a; Kremers et al., 1981). Comparative studies of this kind can be helpful when potential differences between the capacity of embryonic or fetal cells and adult cells of various species for metabolizing xenobiotics are sought.

### 5.4.5 "Micromass" culture of dispersed cells from the embryonic limb and lung

On the basis of work performed with cells of chick embryos (Caplan, 1970; Schacter, 1970; Levitt et al., 1975), a method was developed for the study of cartilage formation from limb blastema cells grown at high cell density (Umansky, 1966; Ahrens et al., 1977; Pennypacker et al., 1978b; Solursh et al., 1978). This technique is referred to as micromass, spot, or high density cell culture. Dispersed cells from a number of organ anlagen can be used for this purpose.

Blastema cells from the limbs of 11-day-old mouse embryos are disintegrated with trypsin and the dispersed cells cultured in a drop of culture medium in a Petri dish. At the time of initiation of the culture, there is no or little indication of the formation of cartilaginous structures in the anlage. After two days in culture, nodules of cartilage form *in vitro*. This system has been used extensively in several laboratories, and the effect of a variety of chemical agents on cartilage formation has been investigated (Hassel et al., 1978; Pennypacker et al., 1978a,b; Lewis et al., 1978; Flint, 1980; Merker et al., 1980a,b). The culture system has a major disadvantage; it is not possible to study typical morphogenetic differentiations, only differentiation at the cellular level. However, the advantage of this system is that the technique is easy and results are obtained after a comparatively short period.

Merker and his group established a system in which it is possible to observe the morphogenetic differentiation processes in lung cells (Merker et al., 1981). The tissue of a lung anlage from a 14-day-old mouse embryo is disintegrated with trypsin and collagenase and the cells cultured at high density in a drop of culture medium in a Petri dish. Budding with structures resembling embryonic lung tissues, can be obtained in culture. Abnormal development has also been studied using this system (Zimmermann et al., 1981).

### 5.4.6 Studies with non-embryonic tissues

It may be asked whether it is feasible to use non-embryonic tissues for evaluating the possible embryotoxic effects of chemicals. Basic processes such as cell-cell interactions, cell migrations, differentiation processes, and proliferation processes, can be used as end points, as these are certainly involved in embryonic development. Systems suggested so far include the investigation of aggregation phenomena with cells of mammalia (Moscona & Moscona, 1952) or lower invertebrates such as hydra (Johnson, 1981), the investigation of cell-cell interactions as studied by the attachment of cells to lectin-coated surfaces (Braun et al., 1979, 1982), and the possibility of studying induction processes using hormones or drugs. The use of teratocarcinoma cells, which are pluripotent cells capable of many types of embryonic differentiation, might also be considered (Stevens, 1967; Graham, 1977; Martin, 1978).

The regeneration of the tail of the *Xenopus* larvae or of the crested newt has been suggested as a model for the evaluation of the teratogenic potential of drugs. The biology of this regeneration has been well investigated (e.g., Lüscher, 1946, 1955; Gebhardt & Faber, 1966; Thornton, 1968; Neukomm, 1969; Tsonis & Eguchi, 1980) and possible means of interfering with this regeneration have been explored. It has been found possible to induce abnormal regeneration in this system with thalidomide and some of its teratogenic and non-teratogenic derivatives (Bazzoli et al., 1977). There are no systematic studies on the use of such systems in routine testing for embryotoxicity.

# 6. HUMAN RISK ASSESSMENT

## 6.1 Introduction

Human risk assessment is intended to provide an estimate of the potential for human disease, and of exposure levels for protecting human health. The dose-effect data from human epidemiological and/or environmental animal studies are essential for human risk evaluation. When coupled with estimates of actual exposure levels, they can be used to estimate the probability (magnitude of the likelihood) of an effect in the exposed population. Such a hazard assessment[a] requires a quantitative evaluation of exposure for each sub-population at risk. Since the assessment of hazard for sub-populations necessarily relies on the level and type of exposure specific to each circumstance, hazard assessment is not discussed in this document.

Direct observations in human beings obviously provide the best information for assessing human risk. These data, however, are rarely available and may often be difficult to interpret, particularly with respect to the timing and level of exposure. Given these factors, scientists most often rely on observations from laboratory animal studies to estimate potential human risks associated with environmental exposures.

Most experience with risk assessment has been in the area of carcinogenesis, although methods are being developed for assessing risk for other health endpoints (EPA, 1976; Albert et al., 1977; IRLG, 1979; EPA, 1980; EPA, 1982; NAS, 1983). The assessment of human risk from prenatally-induced toxicity presents particular problems, which are described in this chapter. In general, the risk assessment comprises two steps: (a) a qualitative assessment of the biomedical data to determine the likelihood that the chemical may pose human risks of prenatally-induced toxicity, and (b) on the assumption that the chemical is capable of causing such adverse effects, a quantitative estimate or prediction of the dose-effect relationships in human beings, to provide the basis for recommending safe exposure levels and for further assessing the potential hazard to sub-populations exposed to the chemical at various levels.

The first step (i.e., qualitative assessment) relies on observations in human beings and laboratory animals together

---

[a] In this context, the term "hazard assessment" is used to indicate the likelihood that a chemical will cause an adverse health effect (injury) under the conditions in which it is produced or used (WHO, 1978).

with other pertinent supporting data. Taking a weight-of-evidence approach, observations in human beings, backed up by animal studies, provide the most convincing evidence that a chemical is capable of causing adverse effects in developing progeny. In the absence of human data, however, observations in laboratory animals must be relied on. The best animal evidence is provided by replicated results in laboratory animals and results in multiple species. Experimental animal data of a more limited nature may contribute some evidence of potential adverse human effects provided the design and conduct of the study is adequate; although the data for each chemical must be evaluated independently. In an assessment of these data, the nature, severity, and extent of the biological responses should be considered together with other data that may have a bearing on the overall evaluation. These include pharmacokinetic parameters, cytotoxicity, other toxic endpoints, structure-activity relationships, maternal toxicity, and information from short-term non-mammalian and in vitro tests.

The second step, that of quantitatively estimating the dose-effect relationship for human beings, generally requires extrapolation from higher doses, where effects have been observed in human beings or in laboratory animals, to lower doses to which human beings may be exposed in the environment. A dose-response relationship, observed in human beings is more readily interpretable for low-dose extrapolation than animal data. Very often, however, observations in human beings are not accompanied by very precise estimates of the magnitude and duration of exposure. In the absence of such data, experimental animal data may be used to extrapolate dose-effect relations for human beings. For this, it is usually necessary to fit some shape to the dose-effect curve outside the observed range, with a view to extrapolating adverse effects observed at higher doses in experimental studies to possible effects that might occur at lower human exposure. The shape of the dose-effect curve should be justified, if possible, on the basis of mechanisms of action. It is also necessary to compensate for the biological, especially pharmacokinetic, differences between animals and human beings. Although a variety of mathematical models have been suggested for extrapolation involving other toxic manifestations, e.g., carcinogenicity (Brown, 1980; Anderson & CAG, in press), their applicability for predicting adverse health effects in progeny following exposure during pregnancy has not been justified. In the absence of a biological justification for applying mathematical extrapolation models to these biological data, safety factors are being used to recommend safe levels of exposure. Various factors involved in data interpretation for the purpose of human risk assessments are discussed in sections 6.2 and 6.3.

## 6.2 Interpreting Laboratory Animal Studies

For qualitative risk assessment purposes, positive results in laboratory animals may provide substantial evidence that the agent may be a potential human teratogen. However, animal studies must be interpreted in the light of the adequacy of the study and the nature and extent of the responses, together with all other biological information that might have a bearing on the weight-of-evidence to establish potential human teratogenicity.

The primary basis for using animal bioassay systems to predict prenatally-induced toxicity in human beings is that almost all of the 15-20 known or suspected human chemical teratogens give positive results in animal bioassay systems (Schardein, 1983; Shepard, 1983). However, many agents shown to induce developmental toxicity in laboratory animals have not been clearly associated with human effects. Factors such as interspecies differences, and the use of very high doses, often causing toxic effects in the dam, in experimental animal studies compared with the low levels to which human beings are exposed, may account for this. It is possible that most agents that produce teratogenic effects in laboratory animals would also be shown to affect human beings, if the methods for detection were sufficiently sensitive and the human exposures were high enough.

Several approaches have been proposed for classifying the qualitative evidence for developmental toxicity. For example, Neubert et al. (1980) have proposed that agents that cause developmental toxicity should be classified as inducing non-specific or specific effects. Non-specific effects can be induced by almost any agent, if the doses are high enough. These effects include weight reduction, developmental retardation, and embryo-mortality. Such effects may often be caused by maternal toxicity and may, therefore, warrant different quantitative approaches. If maternal toxicity is the cause of the fetal effect, then the extrapolation of experimental data is carried out according to the methods used in adult toxicity. Also lower safety factors are often used for such agents. On the other hand, agents that cause specific effects do so by interfering with some stage of fetal development, independent of maternal toxicity. For specific effects, any extrapolation must be related to the fetal effect and be based on the mechanisms of action, if possible, and safety factors higher than those for non-specific effects should be used. Similar use of different safety factors for different classes of effects has been proposed by Khera (in press). One of the difficulties associated with using any categorization scheme is that some chemicals may not fall clearly into any one category.

The adequacy of animal data depends in part on experimental conditions. The route, temporal pattern, and duration of exposure for experimental studies should simulate those of man for use in performing risk assessments. Sometimes it might be advisable to test impure chemicals or chemical formulations to which man is exposed.

Despite widespread interest in short-term non-mammalian and in vitro techniques, pregnant mammals are today the only accepted test systems for predicting human disease. Currently, some short-term test systems offer promise for elucidating the mechanisms of action of embryotoxic agents and some may also be useful for providing supporting information for interpreting animal bioassay studies.

### 6.2.1 Endpoints

A wide variety of responses characterize developmental toxicity. Spontaneous abortion, intrauterine death, prematurity, low birth weight, birth defects, and postnatal manifestation following prenatal insults are effects of abnormal human and animal reproduction. Even offspring that seem perfectly normal at birth may be afflicted with some degree of mental retardation or with transplacentally-induced infertility (Khera & Ruddick, 1973) and cancer later in life. At present, most of the evidence regarding these types of delayed toxicity is derived from studies on animals, though a few examples have come to light in human beings. These are that prenatal exposure to diethyl stilboestrol impaired fertility in male and female offspring and induced vaginal cancer in female offspring (Herbst et al., 1979b) and prenatal exposure to methyl mercury induced cerebral palsy in offspring (Reuhl & Chang, 1979). Thus, risk assessment is complicated by the various outcomes of altered development that need to be considered. Mechanisms of action may differ for these different endpoints; therefore characterization of dose-effect curves, particularly at low levels of exposure, to quantitatively assess human risk for different disease endpoints is complex.

The various endpoints of developmental toxicity can occur spontaneously or be induced. Altered growth consists of reduced fetal weight, which is widely recognized, and increased fetal weight which is less recognized. Structural variations include changes of a permanent nature i.e., extra rib, absent vertebral segment, retarded ossification, precocious ossification, and open ductus arteriosus. The role of minor structural deviations relative to more obvious forms of developmental toxicity in animals and human beings has not received sufficient attention to determine their relative significance in human risk assessment (Khera, 1981).

### 6.2.2 Interspecies variations

Even among laboratory species, the embryotoxic and teratogenic responses to the same chemical may vary markedly. Such variations in response complicate the extrapolation of laboratory animal data to man, because it is not known which is the best animal model. Interspecies differences are presumably due to differences in the intrinsic sensitivity of embryonic and fetal processes to chemical perturbation, the rate and stage of embryogenesis, and various toxicokinetic factors (Neubert & Chahoud, 1983; Khera, in press).

There is also a difference in the background for developmental abnormalities between some laboratory animal species and human beings. For example, the preimplantation and early postimplantation losses in rats are low, less than 10% (Perraud, D., 1976; Fritz, H. et al., 1978; Frohberg, 1977), while the fetal wastage in human beings may be as high as 50% (section 3.1.1.1). Human beings have an apparent mechanism to naturally abort, particularly if the fetus is abnormal. At present, not enough is known to account for these differences in predicting potential human disease.

If a teratogen acts by means of the same biochemical mechanism in the animal model and in man, then the concentration of the chemical at the target site is an important determinant of the susceptibility of the species. In turn, the concentration of the chemical at the target cell is determined by pharmacokinetic variables. By modelling pharmacokinetic constants in the test species and man, it may be possible to predict the incidence of teratogenicity based on maternal blood concentrations.

The differences in toxicokinetics make it almost impossible to extrapolate data from rodents to man with any certainty (Khera, 1976). Nau et al. (1981) demonstrated that, with the use of "minipumps", concentrations similar to the therapeutic concentrations obtained in human beings can be obtained in mice for valproic acid. Such methods may aid an evaluation of teratogenic effects.

Pharmacokinetic models may greatly aid in assessing the human risk associated with exposure to potential teratogens. These procedures, however, must be perfected and validated. In the future, computer models based on well-validated mechanisms, structure-activity relationships, pharmacokinetic data, *in vitro* data, and whole animal models should greatly enhance the reliability of data extrapolation from laboratory animals to man.

### 6.2.3 Statistical limitations

Although many variables are controlled in well-conducted animal tests, there remains the major problem of the statistical limitation of the study. A basic aspect of toxicology is the dose-response relationship relating the incidence of a specific effect induced by a chemical to increasing exposure levels. The incidence of an effect and the size of the study population are important in determining the sensitivity of the study. Because the underlying mechanisms may be different, it is advisable, in principle, to evaluate dose-effect relationships for all prenatally-induced toxic effects, separately. When considering effects as completely separate entities, it must be recognized that the relevant dose-range for that effect may be severely restricted. If the endpoints studied are restricted to "all or none", such as low frequency events of malformations or abortions, then the power of statistical tests in studies of conventional dimensions is often extremely poor. Because a single effect in prenatal toxicity may often be modulated and obscured by other effects of toxicity, such an approach can frequently prove unsatisfactory. In such a case, the evaluation of compiled data concerning several effects may be necessary, although not completely justified. For the purposes of interpretation of animal data for predicting potential human disease, the dose-effect relationship of the most sensitive effect has the greatest significance.

Statistical tests should be used as a guide and not as a substitute for biological judgement. Before statistical significance can be transformed to toxicological relevance, the result must make biological sense and the same applies to "non-significant" results.

Since by using fetus or litter as the statistical unit, important data may be lost, it is advisable to report effects based both on the number of litters and on the total number of fetuses observed (Neubert & Dilmann, 1972). Statistical methods for combining fetal and litter data for evaluating chemically-induced effects have been described (Snedecor & Cochran, 1967; Sokal & Rohlf, 1969; Haseman & Kupper, 1979; Haseman & Hogan, 1975).

### 6.2.4 Quantitative risk assessment

Since there is no universally-accepted mathematical model for extrapolating embryotoxic including teratogenic effects below the observed dose-effect range, safe levels of exposure for human beings have been estimated by applying a safety factor to the no-observed-teratogenic-effect level (Lehman et al., 1954; FDA, 1974; EPA, 1975; NAS, 1977; Faber, 1980;

ACGIH, 1981; Khera, 1984). Usually, large safety factors are used, because it is not possible to accurately characterize synergistic or antagonistic factors that may occur in human beings through exposure to a combination of chemicals in the ambient environment. Khera (in press) compared the quantitative dose-effect data available in the literature for embryotoxic effects in human beings and animals. Using crude estimates, the ratios between the lowest doses of several drugs reported in literature to have produced adverse effects in human progeny and the lowest reported embryotoxic doses in various animal species varied between 1 and 400.

A number of statistical (tolerance) models, such as probit, logit, and Weibul, which were developed for other toxicological endpoints, might also be used to describe teratogenic dose-response relationships. Other mechanistic models such as the multi-hit and multi-stage models have been specifically developed for the carcinogenic response (Mantel & Schreiderman, 1975; Chaud & Hoel, 1974; Brown, 1980; Krewski & Van Ryzin, 1981). The tolerance models were developed on the basis of the notion that each individual in the population possesses a tolerance to the test compound. If dose D does not exceed the tolerance for an individual, then there will be no effect on that individual; while a dose exceeding the tolerance will result in a positive response. The probability that the individual selected at random will respond at a dose D is given by,

$$P = f(D) = \Pr[\text{tolerance} \leq D]$$

The probit model is obtained when the tolerance is considered as a random variable, and follows a log normal distribution. Logit and Weibul models are obtained when the tolerance is assumed to follow logistic or extreme value distribution, respectively. The logit, like the probit model, has an S-shaped dose-response curve that is symmetric about the 50% response point. The logit curve approaches the zero response more slowly than the probit curve, leading to a higher response rate for a given dose in the low-dose region (Brown, 1980).

All these statistical (tolerance) models and the mechanistic models will probably fit teratological dose-response data in the observed range reasonably closely; but would be expected to diverge substantially in the low-dose region. Since the risk estimates obtained at low doses from both the statistical (tolerance) models and the mechanistic models are expected to cover a wide spectrum at low doses, they could be used to define a range of risk estimates at a given exposure level. The primary reason for believing that such a risk range is plausible is based on the hypothesis that most biological effects have a dose-response curve in the low-dose range that is concave upwards. If this is also true for teratogens, then the above models would establish a broad risk range for a given low dose exposure. However, low-dose extrapolation for teratogens is largely an uninvestigated field. Only with knowledge of the mechanisms of action, can an appropriate extrapolation model be selected for better describing risk at low doses for embryotoxic agents including teratogens.

Probit models have been proposed as an extrapolation model to determine safe human exposure levels (Mantel & Bryan, 1961; Weil, 1972). Probit models have also been used to compare the relative teratogenicity of different chemicals in a specific animal species (Fabro et al., 1981) and to fit experimental data in an observed dose-effect range (Neubert et al., 1973).

Biddle (1978) studied the potential of cortisone and 6-aminonicotinamide to induce cleft palate in a variety of inbred and hybrid mouse strains using a probit model. For both compounds, a separate family of parallel dose-effect curves was derived from the experimental data generated by studying the different genotypes. Parallel dose-effect curves were assumed to suggest a common mechanism of teratogenicity. Biddle concluded that when dose-effect curves for the different strains have the same slope, the ratios of estimated $ED_{50}$s provide the most reasonable measure of relative strain sensitivity. Hogan & Hoel (1982) pointed out the limitations of this approach. Their main criticism was that, because approximately parallel dose-response curves for different strains of mice were restricted to the experimental dose range, it was not possible to know whether they would persist in the low-dose region, near the origin of the curve.

An attempt to ascertain whether a "threshold" exists in prenatal toxicity and whether embryotoxic agents may be grouped in different categories in this respect was made by Jusko (1972). Using a mathematical model and a graphing procedure, he suggested that embryotoxic substances might be grouped in two mechanists categories: agents that show a "threshold" and others that do not, with implications for low-dose extrapolation. Although the method suffers from the common difficulty of having to project data in the low-dose range, the approach seems worthy of consideration with appropriate experimental data.

In any attempt to extrapolate animal data, the possible contribution of maternal toxicity to the toxic effects in the fetus must be considered, because most chemicals could damage the fetus by this mechanism, if exposure were high enough (Martson & Shepelskaja, 1982, 1983). In recent studies, attempts have been made to quantify the toxic effects on the mother and the embryo and to associate dose-response relationships of the various parameters. From the data, it is possible to calculate indices, derived by comparing doses for the maternal toxic responses with the dose producing embryotoxic effects, including teratogenic effects (Murphy, 1965; Chaube & Murphy, 1968; Johnson, 1981; Vergieva, 1981, 1982; Bass et al., 1982; Fabro et al., 1981, 1982; Platzek et al., 1982). In some situations, these indices are being used to classify the relative hazard of environmental agents such as pesticides (Kalojanova, 1982) and to estimate safe levels for water pollutants (Vitvitskaja et al., 1980; Korolev & Agareva, 1983).

### 6.3 Interpretation of Human Data for Risk Assessment

Human data are the most reliable basis for estimating risks of human disease. These data, however, are difficult to obtain and may be of limited value for risk assessment because of confounding variables common to all epidemiology studies, including difficulties in exposure estimation, high background rates of birth defects in the human population, and wide variation in diagnosing and reporting defects. These factors were discussed in detail in section 3.1 (Human studies). For the purposes of quantitative risk extrapolation, the model that best fits the human dose-effect data in the observed range should be used and extrapolated to lower doses, if possible, on the basis of plausible mechanisms of action. Even negative human data can be useful for comparison with dose-effect relationships and risk levels estimated from animal data, in determining an upper level for possible human risk.

# 7. CONCLUSIONS

In concluding this report, it is worthwhile to return to the questions posed in the introduction to the document:

(a) What is the value of currently used toxicity tests for predicting human risk?

(b) What are the difficulties involved in applying these test results to estimate human health risks and hazards?

(c) Can better testing strategies be developed?

1. Animal tests are valuable in identifying chemicals that can alter morphological and functional development. Extrapolation from such data to man is the principal method of predicting health risks. Prenatally-induced toxicity is identified in animals and its transposition to man depends on essential elements in the experimental design. The species (and strain) of the test animal must be carefully selected, bearing in mind availability, fecundity, and the incidence of spontaneous malformations or variations. A knowledge of toxicokinetic variables, homeostatic mechanism, and ability to adapt to a chemical insult, relative to man, greatly aid in extrapolating laboratory data to man. If a study is properly executed, it is possible to compare fetal and maternal levels of toxicity.

2. A number of difficulties are involved in applying laboratory animal test data to estimate human risks. They become all the more pronounced, when attempting a quantitative risk assessment. Animal studies usually involve healthy animals; food and water and other environmental factors are controlled; adequate group sizes are possible; and exposure is usually to a single agent. The offspring can be carefully examined at any time. In contrast, an exposed human population varies in genetic constitution, health, diet, and physical environment. In addition, the subjects under study may elect to smoke, consume alcoholic beverages, or take drugs.

Human studies are perhaps the weakest link in the chain of events, necessary to develop and validate means of predicting human risk to a toxic chemical. In epidemiology studies, it is rarely possible to identify the ideal test population and its control; the numbers of individuals in the test group are usually small and the incidence of the effect low and difficult to detect. Toxic effects may be apparent at birth or manifest later during postnatal life. Therefore, few environmental chemicals have been shown to be toxic to the human fetus. However, when collecting human epidemiological data, data on accidental exposure and other evidence of human hazards is emphasized. Toxicokinetic data can sometimes be obtained on human beings occupationally or accidentally exposed to chemicals. Quantitative data on human exposures are essential, both in conducting human studies to establish dose-response relationships and for the estimation of risks to sub-populations exposed to various levels of environmental agents.

3. There is no question that better testing strategies could be developed in both laboratory animals and human studies. Topics that deserve emphasis include comparative toxicokinetic studies to enable interspecies comparison of test results and extrapolation to man; a better understanding of the genetic, molecular, and cellular processes that are the targets for toxic chemicals, which disturb them and cause dysfunction; short-term tests in which enzymes, cells, organs, and embryos in culture are used as well as sub-mammalian species; and studies on effects of prenatal chemical exposure on neurobehavioural development and on cancer incidence.

4. Though data on the molecular biology of development and morphogenetics is also increasing, information and understanding of crucial development processes is still rudimentary. Nevertheless, available data seem to suggest that the biological mechanisms underlying normal development are similar and that interspecies differences are often only temporal in nature. The disciplines of genetics, and molecular and cellular biology provide the experimental and clinical scientist with tools to detect altered genes or genetic regulation. A molecular explanation should be sought for every endpoint induced by chemicals in experimental animals.

5. Considerable scientific activity is concerned with the development of short-term tests. They are useful research tools for investigating the processes underlying normal and abnormal development. However, the Task Group was of the opinion that, with the present state of knowledge, short-term tests cannot replace whole animal-testing procedures for assessing risk to human subjects. Short-term tests should be further developed to provide information to support data obtained in whole experimental animal studies, to provide a basis for selecting chemicals for further testing, and to develop models for possible correlation with results from whole animal tests.

6. Morphological defects at birth represent only a part of the effects produced by prenatal toxicity. The process of development during its various stages is also susceptible to chemically-induced adverse effects, manifested during postnatal life. These could involve every tissue and organ system and function, such as the immune system, reproductive capacity, neurobehavioural function. Transplacental carcinogenesis belongs to this category.

Although the importance of the potential effects of prenatal exposure to chemicals on postnatal development is acknowledged, there are, at present, no generally agreed testing strategies for the evaluation of the postnatal manifestation of such effects. However, it may be worth investigating the relative adult versus fetal sensitivity to chemicals to which many pregnant women have been, or are, unavoidably exposed. As a primary task, compounds that are suspected of being human carcinogens (IARC, 1982), should be tested for transplacental carcinogenicity.

7. For qualitative risk assessment, results from human studies, backed up by animal studies, provide the strongest evidence that a chemical is toxic to the developing progeny, if the mother is exposed during pregnancy. In the absence of human studies, positive results in animal studies provide evidence that the agent is potentially toxic for the developing fetus, although the importance of carefully evaluating each individual study and all related biomedical evidence in completing the qualitative risk assessment is essential. Categorizing of embryotoxic effects into specific fetal effects and non-specific effects is useful for establishing safety guidance.

8. At present, the statistical (tolerance) and mechanistic extrapolation models that have been designed for extrapolating high dose-effect data to lower doses for cancer and other toxicological endpoints, remain largely uninvestigated for teratogens. Use of these models for teratogenic extrapolation, as a general matter, can only establish broad risk ranges associated with low-dose levels of exposure, unless there is some indication of the mode of action and some rational basis for extrapolating from the test species to man.

## 8. RECOMMENDATIONS FOR FUTURE ACTIVITIES

The Task Group was of the opinion that, though progress has been made in the evaluation of risks for progeny following prenatal exposure to chemicals, very little information on the mechanisms by which adverse effects are produced has been forthcoming. The Group believed that the following recommendations, if carried out, would enhance the predictive value of the present approaches:

1. In the areas of genetics, and cellular and molecular biology, a number of new techniques have been developed. These involve: cell fusion, cellular migration, interaction and pattern formation, monoclonal antibodies, embryo transfer, whole chromosome and/or gene transfer, production and use of chimeric animals, gene isolation, *in vitro* mutagenesis, and general recombinant-DNA methods. Such techniques should be applied to determine the underlying *mechanisms in normal and abnormal development* with a view to understanding and controlling chemically-induced congenital abnormalities.

2. The following improvements in the design and conduct of *human studies* are recommended:

   (a) Collaborative international epidemiological studies, using standard techniques and quantitative assessments of exposure, should be performed. The information will be useful in the study of the responses of different sub-populations to particular chemicals. These studies can also provide dose-response data to validate animal models for human risk assessment.

   (b) Registries monitoring congenital malformations and pediatric tumours should be expanded to increase the number of participating countries. Data on the frequency and geographical distribution of malformations and infant neoplasms should be published regularly.

   (c) Monitoring of occupational health should include complete reproductive and exposure data of workers. Special risk groups should be studied for pregnancy outcomes. Pregnancy wastage, including spontaneous abortions, intrauterine deaths, and the more subtle effects that occur prenatally or develop postnatally, must also be considered.

(d) Relationships, if any, between structural defects and biochemical and/or functional defects, and fetal loss should be investigated.

(e) Methods should be established to diagnose so-called "minor abnormalities" in the general population and in risk groups.

3. In order to make the animal embryotoxicity studies more meaningful for extrapolation to human safety, the following suggestions are made:

(a) It has been suggested that 3.5% of all human malformations are associated with the ill health and disease conditions of the mother (Kalter & Warkany, 1983). However, in animal studies, the role of maternal toxicity in the induction of fetal anomalies and embryotoxicity needs clarification. Such a clarification would be extremely helpful in the embryo/fetal evaluation of chemicals and extrapolation of human safety from animal data.

(b) The role of maternal, placental, and fetal factors in activating or detoxifying environmental chemicals in different animal species and man should be clarified.

(c) The significance of different kinds of experimentally-induced gross structural abnormalities for a human risk assessment must be determined by well-designed studies.

(d) Studies should be designed with a view to defining target cells or receptors in the fetus that are specific for teratogens.

(e) Since human beings are usually exposed to a variety of chemicals, studies on the treatment of pregnant animals with a combination of two or more chemicals are suggested.

(f) In view of increasing knowledge, the design and interpretation of animal studies should be periodically appraised by an international group of experts.

4. Attention must be directed to the entire spectrum of developmental toxicity including postnatal manifestations in human and animal studies. Test methods must be

developed to monitor neonates and young children of mothers exposed to chemicals during pregnancy, for functional abnormalities. This should include evaluation of neurobehavioural effects, the immune and endocrine systems, and of xenobiotic metabolism, preferably with non-invasive methods. The background data for these functions must be established.

5. Additional effort is needed to evaluate neurobehavioural tests for routine use in developmental toxicology. Attention should be given to:

    (a) selection of chemicals that can be used as positive controls;

    (b) identification of the most suitable tests and periods during postnatal development;

    (c) development of procedures for the early detection of latent neurotoxic effects; and

    (d) better understanding of basic mechanisms underlying neurobehavioural effects.

6. The following research needs were recognized in the area of transplacental carcinogenicity:

    (a) Fetal exposure to carcinogens in animal studies has been reported to increase susceptibility to tumour induction following further exposure, postnatally, to various carcinogens or promoting agents (section 4.4). Verification of these results is needed.

    (b) Results of a few animal studies have suggested that chemical exposure of the parent generation can be followed by an increased incidence of tumours in subsequent generations (section 4.4). This phenomenon should be explored further.

    (c) Animal models with a comparatively long pregnancy should be investigated to estimate the susceptibility of the embryo/fetus to transplacental carcinogens at various stages of development.

7. (a) Short-term tests should be further developed to provide information on embryotoxic mechanisms and to determine their use for selecting chemicals for further animal testing;

(b) Short-term tests that show promise for chemical selection should be validated using the principles provided in section 5. An international meeting to discuss validation methods is needed. The sensitivity and susceptibility of any technique considered for use in short-term selection tests must be established taking into account results from <u>in vivo</u> studies.

8. (a) <u>Toxicokinetic models</u> should be developed in order to compare toxic effects among species, based on the amount of chemical present in the maternal blood, various tissues, or even at receptor sites of the dam or embryo. These data are needed because a satisfactory risk assessment for human beings can never be based solely on the doses administered to animals and the human exposure levels. Toxicokinetics, and homeostatic and adaptive factors largely account for differences in response. Finally, these data are needed to establish a better understanding of the mechanisms of action as a basis for qualitative risk extrapolation.

(b) Research is needed to (i) generate basic biological information that will provide a more rational scientific basis for the proper application of safety factors for estimating "safe levels" of exposure; and (ii) develop the biological basis for selecting appropriate mathematical models. These methods are germane to <u>extrapolation from high doses in animal studies to low exposure levels in human beings</u>, in order to estimate the magnitude of effect in human beings.

9. <u>Priority for testing</u> should be high for chemicals: (i) that show an increased potential for altering development by affecting genetic, molecular, or cellular processes; (ii) that show structural similarities to known human teratogens; and (iii) to which women of child-bearing age will probably be exposed.

## 9. EXPLANATION OF TERMS USED IN THE DOCUMENT

This section explains the meanings of certain terms as used in this document. These meanings are not necessarily valid for other purposes.

Conceptus

All products of conception derived from and including the fertilized ovum at any time during pregnancy, including the embryo or fetus and embryonic membranes.

Congenital malformation

A permanent structural abnormality present at birth.

Critical period

A particular developmental phase during which a morphogenetic system is especially vulnerable (e.g., neurulation, fusion of the facial swellings, elevation of palatal shelves).

Developmental toxicity

Any adverse effect induced prior to attainment of adult life. This is a new term and includes effects induced or manifested in the embryonic or fetal period and those induced or manifested postnatally (before sexual maturity).

Embryo/fetotoxicity

Any toxic effect on the conceptus resulting from prenatal exposure, including structural or functional abnormalities or postnatal manifestation of such effects.

Embryonic period

The period from conception to the end of major organogenesis. Generally, the organ systems are identifiable at the end of this period.

Fetal period

The period from the end of embryogenesis to the completion of pregnancy.

Poor pregnancy outcome

A term used to describe the failure of a pregnancy to produce viable, biologically normal offspring. It covers all adverse effects: fetal death (including abortion), intra-uterine growth retardation and abnormal development.

Pregnancy dating and conceptional age

Throughout the text, Day 0 is considered to be the first day of pregnancy. In human beings, gestational age (date from first day of last menstrual period) and conceptional age (date from conception) may be used. In this document, conceptional age has been adopted .

Prenatally-induced abnormality

Any structural, functional, or biochemical deviation from the norm, initiated prenatally, that can be detected during prenatal or postnatal life.

Sensitive period

A developmental phase during which differentiating cells become susceptible to a given toxic agent. The period may not be related to critical morphogenetic periods, but may be related to the appearance of specific receptors (e.g., for glucocorticoids).

Teratogen[a]

An agent which when administered prenatally induces permanent abnormalities in structure.

Teratogenicity[a]

A type of embryo/fetotoxicity that is restricted to permanent structural abnormalities produced by prenatal exposure to toxic agents.

---

[a] "Teratogen" and "Teratogenicity" as agreed by the Task Group are used here in the traditional sense derived from Greek word "teratas". They refer to a particular case of embryotoxic effect demonstrated by structural malformation detectable by the present routinely used methods (Section 3.2). The Group recognized that these meanings differ from those used by other bodies.

REFERENCES

ABEL, E.L. (1980) Smoking during pregnancy; a review of effects on growth and development of offspring. Hum. Biol., 52: 593-625.

ACGIH (1981) American Conference on Governmental Industrial Hygienists, TLD for chemical substances and physical agents and the work room environment with interded changes for 1981, Cincinnati, Ohio, ACGIH (Publication Office).

ADAMS, J. & BUELKE-SAM, J. (1981) Behavioral assessment of the postnatal animal: testing and methods development. In: Kimmel, C. A. & Buelke-Sam, J., ed. Developmental toxicology, New York, Raven Press, pp. 233-258.

AHRENS, P.B., SOLURSH, M., & REITER, R.S. (1977) Stage-related capacity for limb chondrogenesis in cell culture. Dev. Biol., 60: 69-82.

AKUTA, T. (1979) Effects of rearing conditions on the behavior of mothers and on the later open-field behavior of the offspring in the mouse. Jpn. J. Psychol., 50: 73-81.

ALBERT, R.E., TRAIN, R.E., & ANDERSON, E. (1977) Rationale developed by the Environmental Protection Agency for the assessment of carcinogenic risks. J. Natl Cancer Inst., 58: 1537-1541.

ALDER, S. & ZBINDEN, G. (1977) Methods for the evaluation of physical, neuromuscular and behavioral development of rats in early postnatal life. In: Neubert, D., Merker, H.-J., & Kwasigroch, T. E., ed. Methods in prenatal toxicology, Stuttgart, georg Thieme Publ., pp. 175-185.

ALEXANDROV, V.A. (1968) Blastomogenic effect of dimethylnitrosamine on pregnant rats and their offspring. Nature (Lond.), 218: 280-281.

ALEXANDROV, V.A. (1969) [Transplacental blastomogenic effect of N-nitrosomethylurea on rat offspring.] Vop. Onkol., N4: 55-61 (in Russian).

ALEXANDROV, V.A. (1972) [Effects of N-nitrosomethylurethane on rat embryos.] Vop. Onkol., N7: 59-64 (in Russian).

ALEXANDROV, V.A. (1973) [Teratogenic and transplacental carcinogenic blastomogenic effect of combined treatment with alkylurea and nitrite (endogenous formation of alkylnitrosourea).] [Proceedings of the First Symposium "Carcinogenic N-nitrosocompounds action, synthesis and detection", Tallin,] pp. 84-86 (in Russian).

ALEXANDROV, V.A. (1974) [Embryotoxic, teratogenic and carcinogenic effects of N-nitrosomethylurea in rats.] Vop. Onkol., 12: 76-82 (in Russian).

ALEXANDROV, V.A. (1976) Some results and prospects of transplacental carcinogenesis studies. Neoplasma, 23: 285-299.

ALEXANDROV, V.A. & ANISIMOV, V.N. (1976) [Peculiarities of transplacental effect of N-nitrosomethylurea in persistent oestrus rats.] Vop. Onkol., 11: 98-102 (in Russian).

ALEXANDROV, V.A. & NAPALKOV, N.P. (1976) Experimental study of relationship between teratogenesis and carcinogenesis in the brain of the rat. Cancer Lett., 1: 345-350.

ALEXANDROV, V.A. & NAPALKOV, N.P. (1979) [Transplacental carcinogenic effect on mice after combined administration of amidopyrine and nitrite.] Vop. Onkol., 7: 48-52 (in Russian).

ALEXANDROV, V.A. & NAPALKOV, N.P. (1981) General regularities of transplacaental (prenatal) carcinogenesis. Biol. Res. Pregnancy, 2: 181-187.

ALLEN, R.W. Jr, OGDEN, B., BENTLEY, F.L., & JUNG, A.L. (1980) Fetal hydantoin syndrome, neuroblastoma, and hemorrhagic disease in a neonate. J. Am. med. Assoc., 244: 1464-1465.

ALTMAN, J. & SUDARSHAN, K. (1975) Postnatal development of locomotion in the laboratory rat. Anim. Behav., 23: 896-920.

ALTMAN, J., SUDARSHAN, K., DAS, G.D., MCCORMICK, N., & BARNES, D. (1971) The influence of nutrition on neural and behavioral development: III. Development of some motor, particularly locomotor patterns during infancy. Dev. Psychobiol., 4: 97-114.

AMSEL, A., BURDETTE, D.R., & LETZ, R. (1976) Appetitive learning, patterned alternation and extinction in 10-d-old rats with non-lactating suckling as reward. Nature (Lond.), 262: 816-818.

ANDERSON, E.L. & THE CARCINOGEN ASSESSMENT GROUP OF THE ENVIRONMENTAL PROTECTION AGENCY (in press) Quantitative methods in use to assess cancer risks. Risk analyses.

ANDREW, F.D. & LYTZ, P.S. (1981) Biochemical disturbances associated with developmental toxicity. In: Kimmel, C.A. & Buelke-Sam, J., ed. Developmental toxicology, New York, Raven Press, pp. 145-165.

ARCHER, J. (1973) Tests for emotionality in rats and mice: a review. Anim. Behav., 21: 205-235.

ARMUTH, V. & BERENBLUM, I. (1977) Possible two-stage transplacental liver carcinogenesis in C57BL/6 mice. Int. J. Cancer, 20: 292-295.

AUSTIN, C.R. (1973) Embryo transfer and sensitivity to teratogenesis. Nature (Lond.), 244: 333-334.

AYDELOTTE, M.B. & KOCHHAR, D.M. (1972) Development of mouse limb buds in organ culture: chondrogenesis in the presence of a proline analog, L-azetidine-2-carboxylic acid. Dev. Biol., 28: 191-201.

BARANOVA, L.N. & ALEXANDROV, V.A. (1978) [Peculiarities of transplacental penetration of 7,12-dimethylbenz(a)anthracene in rats, and its distribution in fetus organs as studied by spectrofluorescent method.] Bull. exp. Biol., 10: 477-479 (in Russian).

BARRACH, H.J. & NEUBERT, D. (1980) Significance of organ culture techniques for evaluation of prenatal toxicity. Arch. Toxicol., 45: 161-187.

BARRACH, H.J., RAUTENBERG, M., TAPKEN, S., NEUBERT, D. (1975) Some biochemical characteristics of mouse limb buds differentiating in organ culture. In: Neubert, D. & Merker, H.-J., ed. New approaches to the evaluation of abnormal embryonic development, Stuttgart, Georg Thieme Publ., pp. 114-132.

BARRACH, H.J., BAUMANN, I., & NEUBERT, D. (1978) The applicability of in vitro systems for the evaluation of the significance of pharmacokinetic parameters for the induction of an embryotoxic effect. In: Neubert, D., Merker, H.-J., Nau, H., & Langman, J., ed. Role of pharmacokinetics in prenatal and perinatal toxicology, Stuttgart, Georg Thieme Publ., pp. 323-336.

BARRACH, H.J., GRUNDMANN, K., HINZ, N., & FELIES, A. (1980) Immunofluorescent microscopic investigations of intercellular substances during limb development. In: Merker, H.-J., Nau, H., & Neubert, D., ed. Teratology of the limbs, Berlin, Walter de Gruyter Publ., pp. 272-293.

BARRACH, H.J., GRUNDMANN, K., HINZ, N., & FELIES, A. (1981) Comparison of the differentiation of muscle and connective tissue of mouse limb buds in culture and in vivo: a morphological study by indirect immunofluorescence. In: Neubert, D. & Merker, H.-J., ed. Culture techniques. Applicability for studies on prenatal differentiation and toxicity, Berlin, New York, Walter de Gruyter Publ., pp. 135-159.

BASS, R., NEUBERT, D., STÖTZER, H., & BOCHERT, G. (1982) Effects on reproduction and other toxicological endpoints. Quantitative dose-response models in teratogenesis. Presented at the SGOMSEC Workshop on: "Quantitative estimation of risk to human health from chemicals", Rome, 12-16 July, 1982.

BATTAGLIA, F.C. & MESCHIA, G. (1978) Principal substrates of fetal metabolism. Physiol. Rev., 58: 499-527.

BAZZOLI, A.S., MANSON, J., SCOTT, W.J., & WILSON, J.G. (1977) The effects of thalidomide and two analogues on the regenerating forelimb of the newt. J. Embryol. exp. Morphol., 41: 125-135.

BECK, F. (1977) Evaluation of organs (gross organ pathology). In: Neubert, D., Merker, H.-J., & Kwasigroch, T. E., ed. Methods in prenatal toxicology, Georg Thieme Publ., Stuttgart, pp. 103-112.

BECK, F. & GULAMHUSEIN, A.P. (1980a) The contrast between mouse and ferret limb buds in culture - possible advantages of comparing results from a limb culture system with whole embryo explantation. In: Merker, H.-J., Nau, H., Neubert, D., ed. Teratology of the limbs, Berlin, Walter de Gruyter Publ., pp. 117-127.

BECK, F. & GULAMHUSEIN, A.P. (1980b) The effect of sodium salicylate on limb development. In: Merker, H.-J., Nau, H., & Neubert, D., ed. Teratology of the limbs, Berlin, Walter de Gruyter Publ., pp. 393-401.

BENDEK, G. & HAHN, Z. (1981) Effect of amphetamine on the metabolism and incorporation of $^{3}H$-thymidine into DNA of developing rat brain. Dev. Neurosci., 4: 55-65.

BENESOVA, O., RYCHTER, Z., & JELINEK, R., ed. (1979) Evaluation of embryotoxicity, mutagenicity, and carcinogenicity risks in new drugs, Prague, Universita Karlova.

BENIASVILI, D.S. (1978) [Comparative study of action of some carcinogenic compounds inducing transplacental blastomogenesis in rabbits.] Vop. Onkol., 3: 77-83 (in Russian).

BENIRSCHKE, K. (1975) Placental causes of maldevelopment. In: Berry, C.L. & Poswillo, D.E., ed. Teratology: trends and applications, Berlin, Heidelberg, New York, Springer-Verlag, pp. 148-164.

BERRY, C.L. (1981) Congenital malformations. In: Berry, C.L., ed. Paediatric pathology, Berlin, Heidelberg, New York, Springer-Verlag, pp. 67-86.

BERRY, C.L. & POSWILLO, D.E., ed. (1975) Teratology trends and applications, Berlin, Heidelberg, New York, Springer-Verlag.

BIDDLE, F.G. (1978) Use of dose-response relationship to discriminate between the mechanisms of cleft palate induction by different teratogens: an argument for discussion. Teratology, 18: 247-252.

BIGGERS, J.D., MCLAREN, A., & MICHIE, D. (1958) Variance control in the animal house. Nature (Lond.), 182: 77-80.

BIGGERS, J.D., WHITTEN, W.K., & WHITTINGHAM, D.G. (1971) The culture of mouse embryos in vitro. In: Daniel, J. C., ed. Methods in mammalian embryology, San Francisco, Freeman, W. H., pp. 86-116.

BLANKENBURG, G., RAUTENBERG, M., NEUBERT, D. (1980) Ascorbic acid content of limb buds at different stages of mammalian embryonic development. In: Merker, H.-J., Nau, H., Neubert, D., ed. Teratology of the limbs, Berlin, Walter de Gruyter Publ., pp. 183-190.

BLANKENBURG, G., BLUTH, U., & NEUBERT, D. (1981) On the significance of ascorbate and of cysteine on differentiation of limb buds in organ culture. In: Neubert, D. & Merker, H.-J., ed. Culture techniques. Applicability for studies on prenatal differentiation and toxicity, Berlin, New York, Walter de Gruyter Publ., pp. 197-206.

BLOZOVSKI, D. & CUDENNEC, A. (1980) Passive avoidance learning in the young rat. Dev. Psychobiol., 13: 513-518.

BOCHERT, G., PLATZEK, T., & WIESSLER, M. (1981) Comparison of effects on limb development *in vivo* and *in vitro* using methyl(acetoxymethyl)nitrosamine. In: Neubert, D. & Merker, H.-J., ed. *Culture techniques. Applicability for studies on prenatal differentiation and toxicity*, Berlin, New York, Walter de Gruyter Publ., pp. 223-235.

BOLLES, R.C. & WOODS, P.J. (1964) The ontogeny of behaviour in the albino rat. *Anim. Behav.*, *12*: 427-441.

BÖRZSÖNYI, M., PINTER, A., SURJAN, A., & FARKAS, I. (1976) Transplacental induction of lymphomas in Swiss mice by carbendazim and sodium nitrite. *Int. J. Cancer*, *17*: 742-747.

BÖRZSÖNYI, M., TÖRÖK, G., PINTER, A., SURJAN, A., NADASDI, L., & ROLLER, P. (1980) Carcinogenic effect of dinitrosopiperazine in adult Swiss mice and after transplacental or translactional exposure. *Cancer Res.*, *40*: 2925-2927.

BOUE, J., BOUE, A., & LAZAR, P. (1975) Retrospective and prospective epidemiological studies of 1500 karyotyped spontaneous human abortions. *Teratology*, *12*: 11-26.

BOURNIAS-VARDIABASIS, N. & TEPLITZ, R.L. (1982) Use of *Drosophila* embryon cell cultures as an *in vitro* teratogen assay. *Teratog. Carcinog. Mutag.*, *2*: 333-341.

BOYER, C.C. (1953) Chronology of development for the golden hamster. *J. Morphol.*, *92*: 1-38.

BRACHET, A. (1913) Recherches sur le déterminisme héréditaire de l'oeuf des mammifères. Développement *in vitro* de jeunes vésicules blastodermiques du lapin. *Arch. Biol., Paris*, *28*: 447-503.

BRAUN, A.G., EMERSON, D.J., & NICHINSON, B.B. (1979) Teratogenic drugs inhibit tumour cell attachment to lectin-coated surfaces. *Nature (Lond.)*, *282*: 507-509.

BRAUN, A.G., NICHINSON, B.B., & HOROWICZ, P.B. (1982) Inhibition of tumour cell attachment to concavalin A-coated surfaces as an essay for teratogenic agents: approaches to validation. *Teratog. Carcinog. Mutag.*, *2*: 343-354.

BRINKLEY, L.L. (1980) *In vitro* studies of palatal shelf elevation. In: Pratt, R. M. & Christiansen, R. L., ed.

Current research trends in prenatal craniofacial development, New York, Amsterdam, Oxford, Elsevier/North-Holland Publ., pp. 203-220.

BRINSTER, R.L. (1963) A method for in vitro cultivation of mouse ova from two-cell to blastocyst. Exp. Cell Res., 32: 205-208.

BRINSTER, R.L. (1970) In vitro cultivation of mammalian ova. In: Raspé, G., ed. Advances in the biosciences, Oxford, London, Edinburgh, New York, Toronto, Sidney, Paris, Braunschweig, Pergamon Press - Vieweg, Vol. 4, pp. 199-233.

BRONSTEIN, P.M., NEIMAN, H., WOLKOFF, F.D., & LEVINE, M.J. (1974) The development of habituation in the rat. Anim. Learn. Behav., 2: 92-96.

BROWN, C.C. (1980) High dose to low dose extrapolation in animals. Presented at: The Food and Drug Law Institute Symposium on the Practical Applications of Risk Assessment, June 14 (Proceedings in print).

BRUNNER, R.L., MCLEAN, M., VORHEES, C.V., & BUTCHER, R.E. (1978) A comparison of behavioral and anatomical measures of hydroxyurea induced abnormalities. Teratology, 18: 379-384.

BUELKE-SAM, J. & KIMMEL, C.A. (1979) Development and standardization of screening methods for behavioural teratology. Teratology, 20: 17-30.

BUTCHER, R.E. (1976) Behavioral testing as a method for assessing risk. Environ. Health Perspect., 18: 75-78.

CABE, P.A., TILSON, H.A., MITCHELL, C.L., & DENNIS, R. (1978) A simple recording grip strength device. Pharmacol. Biochem. Behav., 8: 101-102.

CAMPBELL, B.A. & COULTER, X. (1976) Neural and physiological preocesses underlying the development of learning and memory. In: Tighe, T. J. & Leaton, R. N., ed. Habituation: perspectives from child development, animal behaviour and neurophysiology, Hillsdale, New Jersey, Lawrence Erlbaum Associates, pp. 129-157.

CAMPBELL, B.A. & MABRY, P.D. (1973) The role of catecholamines in behavioural arousal during ontogenesis. Psychopharmacology, 31: 253-264.

CAMPBELL, B.A. & RASKIN, L.A. (1978) Ontogeny of habituation and sensitization in the rat. In: Spear, N. A. & Campbell, B. A., ed. Ontogeny of learning and memory, Hillsdale, New Jersey, Lawrence Erlbaum, pp. 67-100.

CAMPBELL, B.A. & STEHOUWER, D.J. (1980) Retention of habituation and sensitization in neonatal rats. Behav. Neurol. Biol., 29: 190-202.

CAMPBELL, B.A., LYTLE, L:D., & FIBIGER, H.C. (1969) Ontogeny of adrenergic arousal and cholinergic inhibitory mechanisms in the rat. Science, 166: 635-637.

CANADA, NATIONAL HEALTH AND WELFARE (1973) Method of testing for carcinogenicity, mutagenicity, teratogenicity, Ottawa, NHW Publishing Department, 139 pp.

CAPLAN, A.I. (1970) Effects of the nicotinamide-sensitive teratogen 3-acetylpyridine on chick limb cells in culture. Exp. Cell Res., 62: 341-355.

CARTER, C.O. (1976) Genetics of common single malformations. Br. med. Bull., 32: 21-26.

CHAHOUD, I. & EGGERT, S. (1978) Drug-induced impairment of liver function in the prenatal period. In: Neubert, D., Merker, J.-H., Nau, H., & Langman, J., ed. Role of pharmacokinetics in prenatal and perinatal toxicology, Stuttgart, Georg Thieme Publ., pp. 263-271.

CHAHOUD, I., MICO-GINER, L., & NEUBERT, D. (1975) Some evaluations of effects of prenatal drug treatment on postnatal development. In: Neubert, D. & Merker, H.-J., ed. New approaches to the evaluation of abnormal embryonic development, Stuttgart, Georg Thieme Publ., pp. 502-516.

CHANCE, M.R.A. (1957) The contribution of environment to uniformity. Coll. Pap. Lab. Anim. Bur., 6: 59.

CHANG, M.C. (1949) Effects of heterologous sera on fertilized rabbit ova. J. gen. Physiol., 32: 291-300.

CHATOT, C.L., KLEIN, N.W., PIATEK, J., & PIERRO, L.J. (1980) Successful culture of rat embryos on human serum: use in the detection of teratogens. Science, 207: 1471-1473.

CHAUBE, S. & MURPHY, M.L. (1968) The teratogenic effects of the recent drugs active in cancer chemotherapy. In: Wollam,

D. H. M., ed. Advances in teratology, New York, London, Academic Press, pp. 181-237.

CHAUD, N. & HOEL, D.G. (1974) A comparison of models for determining safe levels of environmental agents. In: Reliability and biometry, statistical analysis of life length, Philadelphia, Penn., SIAM, pp. 681-700.

CIBA FOUNDATION SYMPOSIUM 27 (new series) (1974) Size at birth, Amsterdam, Oxford, New York, Elsevier, Excerpta Medica, North-Holland, Associated Scientific Publishers.

CIOMS (1983) Safety requirements for the first use of new drugs and diagnostic agents in man, Geneva, Council for International Organizations of Medical Sciences.

CLARKSON, S.G., DOERING, J.V., & RUNNER, M.N. (1969) Growth of postimplantation mouse embryos cultured in a serum-supplemented, chemically defined medium. Teratology, 2: 181-186.

CLEGG, D.J. (1979) Animal reproduction and carcinogenicity studies in relation to human safety evaluation. In: Deichmann, W.B., ed. Toxicology and occupational medicine, New York, Amsterdam, Oxford, Elsevier North Holland, pp. 45-59.

CMEA (1982) [Methodological recommendations, protocols, experimental studies for establishment threshold levels of the effect of industrial compounds on reproductive function]. In: Problemi promišlenoi toksikologii, SEV, Postoiannaja komissija po sotrudničestvu v oblasti zdravoohranenija, Moskva, 1982, pp. 58-75 (in Russian).

COCKROFT, D.L. & COPPOLA, P.T. (1977) Teratogenic effects of excess glucose on head-fold rat embryos in culture. Teratology, 16: 141-146.

CONNORS, T.A. (1975) Cytotoxic agents in teratogenic research. In: Berry, C.L. & Poswillo, D.E., ed. Teratology, trends and applications, New York, Springer-Verlag, pp. 49-79.

COOKE, J. (1976) Mathematical models of biological parameters, Thesis, Hatfield Polytechnic, England.

COOKE, J. (1981) Evaluation of data recording methods for statistical testing of behavioural responses in the rat, Thesis, Cranfield Institute, England.

COOPER, H.K., HAUENSTEIN, E., KOLAR, G.F., & KLEIHUES, P. (1978) DNA alkylation and neuro-oncogenesis by 3,3-dimethyl-1-phenyltriazene. Acta neuropathol. (Berlin), 43: 105-109.

COSTELLO, D.P., DAVIDSIN, M.E., EGGERS, A., FOX, M.H., & HENLEY, C. (1957) Methods for obtaining and handling marine eggs or embryos, Wood Hool, USA, Marine Biology Laboratory.

COUNIS, M.F., CHAUDUN, E., & COURTOIS, Y. (1977) DNA synthesis and repair in terminally differentiating embryonic lens cells. Dev. Biol., 57: 47-55.

COYLE, I., WAYNER, M.J., & SINGER, G. (1976) Behavioral teratogenesis: a critical evaluation. Pharmacol. Biochem. Behav., 4: 191-200.

CROCKER, J.F.S. (1973) Human embryonic kidneys in organ culture: abnormalities of development induced by decreased potassium. Science, 181: 1178-1179.

CROCKER, J.F.S. & VERNIER, R.L. (1970) Fetal kidney in organ culture: abnormalities of development induced by decreased amounts of potassium. Science, 169: 485-487.

CULVER, B. & NORTON, S. (1976) Juvenile hyperactivity in rats after acute exposure to carbon monoxide. Exp. Neurol., 50: 80-98.

DANIEL, J.C., Jr (1965) Studies on the growth of 5-day old rabbit blastocysts in vitro. J. Embryol. exp. Morph., 13: 83-95.

DANIEL, J.C., Jr (1968) Oxygen concentrations for culture of rabbit blastocysts. J. Reprod. Fertil., 17: 187-190.

DAVIS, G.J., MCLACHLAN, J.A., & LUCIER, G.W. (1978) The effect of 7,12-dimethylbenz-(a)-anthracene (DMBA) on the prenatal development of gonads in mice. Teratology, 17: 33A.

DAVIS, L.A., SADLER, T.W., & LANGMAN, J. (1981) In vitro development of the heart under influence of retinoic acid. In: Neubert, D. & Merker, H.-J., ed. Culture techniques. Applicability for studies on prenatal differentiation and toxicity, Berlin, New York, Walter de Gruyter Publ., pp. 101-115.

DAVIS, M. (1980) Neurochemical modulation of sensory motor reactivity: acoustic and tactile startle reflexes. Neurosci. Biobehav. Rev., 4: 241-263.

DELAHUNT, C.S. & LASSEN, L.J. (1964) Thalidomide syndrome in monkeys. Science, 146: 1300-1305.

DEARBORN, E.H. (1967) Comparative toxicity of drugs. Fed. Proc., 26: 1075-1077.

DEMEREC, M., ed. (1950) Biology of Drosophila, New York, John Wiley.

DEPPE, U., SCHIERENBERG, E., COLE, T., KRIEG, C., SCHMITT, D., YODER, B., & VON EHRENSTEIN, G. (1978) Cell lineages of the embryo of the nematode Caenorhabditis elegans. Proc. Natl. Acad. Sci. USA, 75: 376-380.

DEWS, P. & WENGER, G. (1979) Testing for behavioural effects of agents. Neurobehav. Toxicol., 1: 119-127.

DIWAN, B.A. & MEIER, H. (1974) Strain and age-dependent transplacental carcinogenesis by 1-ethyl- 1-nitrosourea in inbred strains of mice. Cancer Res., 34: 764-770.

DIXON, R.L. (1982) Potential of environmental factors to affect development in reproductive systems. Fundam. appl. Toxicol., 2: 5-12.

DOERJER, G., DIESSNER, H., BUCHELER, J., & KLEIHUES, P. (1978) Reaction of 7,12-dimethylbenz[a]anthracene with DNA of fetal and maternal rat tissues in vivo. Int. J. Cancer, 22: 288-291.

DRUCKREY, H. (1973) Chemical structure and action in transplacental carcinogenesis and teratogenesis. In: Tomatis, L., Mohr, U., & Davis, W., ed. Transplacental carcinogenesis, Lyons, pp. 45-58, IARC Sci. Publ., No. 4.

DUSEMUND, B. & BARRACH, H.J. (1981) Quantification of collagen types I and II in mouse limbs during differentiation in vitro and in vivo. In: Neubert, D. & Merker, H.-J., ed. Culture techniques. Applicability for studies on prenatal differentiation and toxicity, Berlin, New York, Walter de Gruyter Publ., pp. 161-169.

DYBAN, A.P. (1977) [Theoretical and applied aspects of experimental teratology]. Ontogenesis (Sov. J. Devel. Biol.), 8(6): 582-589 (in Russian).

DYBAN, A.P., SEKIRINA, G.G., & GOLINSKY, G.F. (1976) [Sensitivity to antifolic drug pyrimethamine early mice embryos _in vitro_ and _in vivo_.] _Bull. exp. Biol. Med._, _10_: 47-51 (in Russian).

DYBAN, A.P., SEKIRINA, G.G., & GOLINSKY, G.F. (1977b) [The effect of aminopterin on the preimplantation rat embryos cultivated _in vitro_.] _Ontogenesis (Sov. J. Devel. Biol.)_, _8_: 121-127 (in Russian).

DYBAN, A.P., PUCHKOV, V.F., POPOV, V. B., & GOLINSKY, G. F. (1979) Testing of some chemical environmental pollutants to teratogenicity using mammalian embryos cultivated _in vitro_. _Proceedings of the US-USSR third Joint Symposium on Problems on Environmental Health_, Suzdal, USSR, pp. 300-322.

EBERT, J.D. & MAROIS, M., ed. (1976) _Tests of teratogenicity in vitro_, Amsterdam, New York, Oxford, North Holland Publishing Co.

EDMONDS, D.K., LINDSAY, K.S., MILLER, J.F., WILLIAMSON, E., & WOOD, P.J. (1982) Early embryonic mortality in women. _Fertil. Steril._, _38_: 447-453.

EDWARDS, J.H. (1969) Familial predisposition in man. _Br. med. Bull._, _25_: 58-64.

EDWARDS, R.G. (1980) _Conception in the human female_. London, New York, Academic Press, pp. 573-667, 668-766.

EDWARDS, R.G., BAVISTER, B.D., & STEPTOE, P.C. (1969) Early stages of fertilization _in vitro_ of human oocytes matured _in vitro_. _Nature (Lond.)_, _221_: 632-635.

EGGER, H.J., WITTFOHT, W., & NAU, H. (1978) Identification of diphenylhydantoin and its metabolites, including the dihydrodiol and the catechols in maternal plasma, placenta and fetal tissues of man. In: Neubert, D., Merker, H.-J., Nau, H., & Langman, J., ed. _Role of pharmacokinetics in prenatal and perinatal toxicology_, Stuttgart, Georg Thieme Publ., pp. 483-497.

EIBS, H.G. & SPIELMANN, H. (1977) Preimplantation embryos. Part II: Culture and transplantation. In: Neubert, D., Merker, H.-J., & Kwasigroch, T.E., ed. _Methods in prenatal toxicology_, Stuttgart, Georg Thieme Publ., pp. 221-230.

ELLIS, T.M. (1967) Environmental influences on drug responses in laboratory animals. In: M.L. Conalty, Husbandry of laboratory animals: Proceedings of the 3rd International Symposium, London, Academic Press, 650 pp.

ENDO, H., NODA, H., KINOSHITA, N., INUI, N., & NISHI, Y. (1980) Formation of a transplacental mutagen, 1,3-di(4-sulfamoylphenyl)triazene, from sodium nitrite and sulfanilamide in human gastric juice and in the stomachs of hamsters. J. Natl. Cancer Inst., 65: 547-551.

ERICKSON, B.H. (1967) Radioresponse of the pre-puberal porcine ovary. Intern. J. radiat. Biol., 13: 57-67.

ERICKSON, J.D., COCHRAN, W.M., & ANDERSON, C.E. (1979) Parental occupation and birth defects. A preliminary report. In: Klingberg, M.A. & Weatherall, J.A.C., ed. Epidemiologic methods for detection of teratogens. Contributions to epidemiology and biostatistics. Basel, München, Paris, London, New York, Sydney, S. Karger, pp. 107-117.

EVANS, H.L. (1978) Behavioral assessment of visual toxicity. Environ. Health Perspect., 26: 53-57.

FABER, E. (1980) Problems in the safety evaluation of tissue residues. J. environ. Pathol. Toxicol., 3: 73-79.

FABRO, S., SHULL, G., & BROWN, N.A. (1982) The relative teratogenic index and teratogenic potency: proposed components of developmental toxicity risk assessment. Teratog. Carcinog. Mutag., 2: 61-76.

FABRO, S. (1973) Passage of drugs and other chemicals into the uterine fluids and preimplantation blastocyst. In: Boréus, L.O., ed. Fetal pharmacology, New York, Raven Press Publ., pp. 443-461.

FABRO, S., SHULL, G., & BROWN, N.A. (1981) The relative teratogenic index: an approach to the estimation of teratogenic potency, Research Triangle Park, TCM, Laboratory of Reproductive and Developmental Toxicology, NIEHS.

FAIRBANKS, M.B. & KOLLAR, E.J. (1974) Inhibition of palatal fusion in vitro by hadacidin. Teratology, 9: 169-178.

FANTEL, A.G. (1982) Culture of whole rodent embryos in teratogen screening. Teratog. Carcinog. Mutag., 2: 231-242.

FANTEL, A.G., GREENAWAY, J.C., JUCHAU, M.R., & SHEPERD, T.H. (1979) Teratogenic bioactivation of cyclophosphamide in vitro. Life Sci., 25: 67-72.

FARIS, R.A. & CAMPBELL, T.C. (1983) Long-term effects of neonatal phenobarbital exposure on aflatoxin B1 disposition in adult rats. Cancer Res., 43: 2576-2583.

FDA (1966) Food and Drug Administration: Guidelines for reproduction studies for safety evaluation of drugs for human use, January 1966, US FDA.

FDA (1970) Food and Drug Administration. Advisory Committee on Protocols for Safety Evaluations: Panel on reproduction Report on Reproduction Studies in the Safety Evaluation of Food Additives and Pesticide Residues. Toxicol. appl. Pharmacol., 16: 264-296.

FDA (1974) Food and Drug Administration, Poisonous or deleterious substances in peanuts, evaporated milk, fish, and shellfish. Fed. Reg., 39: 42738-42752.

FECHTER, L.D. (1974) The effects of L-dopa, clonidine, and apomorphine on the acoustic startle reaction in rats. Psychopharmacology, 39: 331-344.

FELL, H.B. & WEISS, L. (1965) The effect of antiserum, alone and with hydrocortisone, on foetal mouse bones in culture. J. exp. Med., 121: 551-560.

FLINT, O.P. (1980) The effects of sodium salicylate, cytosine arabinoside, and eserine sulphate on rat limb buds in culture. In: Merker, H.-J., Nau, H., & Neubert, D., ed. Teratology of the limbs, Berlin, New York, Walter de Gruyter Publ., pp. 325-338.

FLODH, H., MAGNUSSON, G., & MALMFORS, T. (1977) Toxicological studies on ferastral[R], an iron-poly (sorbitol-gluconic acid) complex. Scand. J. Haematol. Suppl., 32: 58-68.

FOX, W.M. (1965) Reflex ontogeny and behavioural development of the mouse. Anim. Behav., 13: 234-241.

FRAŇKOVÁ, S. (1968) Nutritional and psychological factors in the development of spontaneous behaviour in the rat. In: Scrimshaw, N.S. & Gordon, J.E., ed. Malnutrition, learning and behaviour, Cambridge, Massachusetts, MIT Press, pp. 312-322.

FRAŇKOVÁ, S. (1973) Effect of protein-calorie malnutrition on the development of social behavior in rat. Dev. Psychobiol., 6: 33-43.

FRAŇKOVÁ, S. (1977) Drug-induced changes in the maternal behavior of rats. Psychopharmacology, 53: 83-87.

FRAŇKOVÁ, S. & BARNES, R.H. (1968) Effect of malnutrition in early life on avoidance conditioning and behaviour of adult rat. J. Nutr., 96: 485-493.

FRITZ, H., GRAUWILER, J., HUMMLER, H., LINDT, S., & SCHÖN, H. (1978) Collection of control data from teratologic experiments on mice, rats, and rabbits. Arzneim.-Forsch., 28: 1410-1413.

FROHBERG, H. (1977) An introduction to research in teratology. In: Neubert, D., Merker, H.-J., & Kwasigroch, T. E., ed. Methods in prenatal toxicology, Stuttgart, Georg Thieme Publ., pp. 1-13.

GALBRAITH, D.B. & KOLLAR, E.J. (1974) Effects of L-azetidine-2-carboxylic acid, a proline analogue, on the in vitro development of mouse tooth germs. Arch. oral Biol., 19: 1171-1176.

GEBHARDT, D.O.E. & FABER, J. (1966) The influence of aminopterin on limb regeneration in Ambystoma mexicanum. J. Embryol. exp. Morphol., 16: 143-158.

GELŠTEIN, V. I. (1961) [Development of tumours in mouse offspring after exposure to orthoaminoazotoluene.] Vop. Onkol., N10: 58-64 (in Russian).

GEMBERLING, G.A., DOMJAN, M., & AMSEL, A. (1980) Aversion learning in 5-day-old rats: taste-toxicosis and texture-shock associations. J. comp. Physiol. Psychol., 94: 734-745.

GERALL, A.A. & MCCRADY, R.E. (1970) Receptivity scores of female rats stimulated either manually or by males. J. Endocrinol., 46: 55-59.

GIERER, A., BERKING, S., BODE, H., DAVID, C.N., FLICK, K., HANSMANN, G., SCHALLER, H., & TRENKNER, E. (1972) Regeneration of hydra from reaggregated cells. Nature, New Biol., 239: 98-101.

GILL, W.B., SCHUMACHER, G.F.B., BIBBO, M., STRAUS, F.H. II, & SCHOENBERG, H.W. (1979) Association of diethylstilbestrol exposure in utero with cryptorchidism, testicular hypoplasia and semen abnormalities. J. Urol., 122: 36-39.

(INSBURG, J. (1971) Placental drug transfer. Ann. Rev. ]harmacol., 11: 387-408.

·IVELBER, H.M. & DIPAOLO, J.A. (1968) Growth of explanted :ight day hamster embryos in circulating medium. Nature ;Lond.), 220: 1131-1132.

GOERTTLER, K. & LOEHRKE, H. (1976) Diaplacental carcinogenesis: initiation with the carcinogens dimethylbenzanthracene (DMBA) and urethane during fetal life and postnatal promotion with the phorbol ester TPA in a modified 2-stage Berenblum-Mottram experiment. Virchow's Arch., A 372(1): 29-38.

GOLDSTEIN, L.S., SPINDLE, A.I., & PEDERSEN, R.A. (1975) X-ray sensitivity of the preimplantation mouse embryo in vitro. Radiat. Res., 62: 276-287.

GOLUB, N.I., KOLESNIČENKO, T.S., & ŠABAD, L.M. (1974) [Blastomogenic effect of some nitrogen compounds on offspring of mice.] Bull. exp. Biol., 2: 62-65 (in Russian).

GOTH, R. & RAJEWSKY, M.F. (1974) Persistence of 06-ethylguanine in rat-brain DNA: correlation with nervous system-specific carcinogenesis by ethylnitrosourea. Proc. Natl Acad. Sci., USA, 71: 639-643.

GRAHAM, C.F. (1977) Teratocarcinoma cells and normal mouse embryogenesis. In: Sherman, M.J., ed. Concepts in mammalian embryogenesis, USA, MIT Press, pp. 315-395.

GRANT, E.C. & MACKINTOSH, J.H. (1963) Comparison of the social postures of some laboratory rodents. Behaviour, 21: 246-259.

GRANT, L.D. (1976) Research strategies for behavioral teratology studies. Environ. Health Perspect., 18: 85-94.

GRAUWILER, J. & LEIST, K.H. (1977) A schedule for examination of postnatal development in rats. In: Neubert, D., Merker, H.-J., & Kwasigroch, T.E., ed. Methods in prenatal toxicology, Stuttgart, Georg Thieme Publ., pp. 166-174.

GREENBERG, J.H. (1982) Detection of teratogens by differentiating embryonic neural crest cells in culture; evaluation as a screening system. Teratog. Carcinog. Mutag., 2: 319-323.

GREENGARD, O. (1973) Effects of hormones on development of fetal enzymes. Clin. Pharmacol., Ther., 14: 721-726.

GREENGARD, O. (1975a) Cortisol treatment of neonatal rats: Effects on enzymes in kidney, liver and heart. Biol. Neonat., 27: 352-360.

GREENGARD, O. (1975b) Steroids and the maturation of rat tissues. J. steroid Biochem., 6: 639-672.

GROBSTEIN, C. (1956) Trans-filter induction of tubules in mouse metanephrogenic mesenchyme. Exp. Cell Res., 10: 424-440.

GUNBERG, D.L. (1976) In vitro development of postimplantation rat embryos cultured on dialyzed rat serum. Teratology, 14: 65-69.

GÜTHERT, H., JÄCKEL, E.M., & WARZOK, R. (1973) [Carcinogenic action of ethylnitroso urea in rabbits.] Zbl. allg. Pathol. U. Pathol. Anat., 117: 461-471 (in German).

HAGSTROM, B.C., LONNING, S. (1973) The sea urchin egg as a testing object in toxicology. Acta pharmacol. toxicol., 32 (Suppl. 1): 49 pp.

HALES, B.F. (1982) Comparison of the mutagenicity and teratogenicity of cyclophosphamide and its active metabolites, 4-hydroxycyclophosphamide, phosphoramide mustard, and acrolein. Cancer Res., 42: 3016-3021.

HARVEY, E.G. (1956) The American Arbacia and other sea urchins, Princeton University.

HASEMAN, J.K. & HOGAN, M.D. (1975) Selection of the experimental unit in teratology studies. Teratology, 12: 165-171.

HASEMAN, J.K. & KUPPER, L.L. (1979) Analysis of dichotomous response data from certain toxicological experiments. Biometrics, 35: 281-293.

HASSELL, J.R., PENNYPACKER, J.P., & LEWIS, C.A. (1978) Chondrogenesis and cell proliferation in limb bud cell cultures treated with cytosine arabinoside and vitamin A. Exp. Cell Res., 112: 409-417.

HEINONEN, O.P. (1977) Birth defects and drugs in pregnancy, Littleton, Mass., Publishing Sciences Group.

HELLER, C.G. & CLERMONT, Y. (1964) Kinetics of the germinal epithelium in man. Recent Progr. hormone Res., 20: 545-575.

HEMMINKI, K., MUTANEN, P., SALONIEMI, I., & LUOMA, K. (1981) Congenital malformation and maternal occupation in Finland: multivariate analysis. J. Epid. commun. Health, 35: 5-10.

HERBST, A.L., COLE, P., NORUSIS, M.J., WELCH, W.R., & SCULLY, R.E. (1979a) Epidemiologic aspects and factors related to survival in 384 registry cases of clear cell adenocarcinoma of the vagina and cervix. Am. J. Obstet. Gynecol., 135: 876-886.

HERBST, A.L., SCULLY, R.E., & ROBBOY, S.J. (1979b) Prenatal diethylstilbestrol exposure and human genital tract abnormalities. In: Perinatal carcinogenesis, pp. 25-35 (Natl Cancer Inst. Monogr., Vol. 51).

HERKEN, R. & ANSCHÜTZ, M. (1981) Differentiation of embryonic tissues in whole-embryo cultures as compared to the development in vivo. In: Neubert, D. & Merker, H.-J., ed. Culture techniques. Applicability for studies on prenatal differentiation and toxicity, Berlin, New York, Walter de Gruyter Publ., pp. 19-35.

HETEM, S., KOLLAR, E.J., CUTLER, L.S., & YAGER, J.A. (1975) Effect of α,α-dipyridyl on the basement membrane of tooth germs in vitro. J. dent. Res., 54: 783-787.

HICKS, S.P. & D'AMATO, C.J. (1966) Effects of ionizing radiations on mammalian development. In: Woollam, D.H.M., ed. Advances in teratology, London, Lago Press, pp. 195-250.

HIGURASHI, M., IIJIMA, K., ISHIKAWA, N., HOSHINA, H., & WATANABE, N. (1979) Incidence of major chromosome aberrations in 12 319 newborn infants in Tokyo. Hum. Genet., 46: 163-172.

HINEGARDUER, R.T. (1967) Echinoderms. In: Wilt, F.H. & Wessels, N.K., ed. Methods in developmental biology, T.Y. Cromwell, pp. 139-155.

HOGAN, M.D. & HOEL, D.G. (1982) Extrapolation to man. In: Hayes, A.W., ed. Principles and methods of toxicology, New York, Raven Press, pp. 711-731.

HOLTZER, H., ABBOTT, J., & LASH, J. (1958) On the formation of multinucleated myotubes. Anat. Rec., 131: 567-568.

HÖRSTADIUM, S. (1973) Experimental embryology of echinoderms, Oxford, Clarendon Press.

HSU, Y.C. (1979) In vitro development of individually cultured whole mouse embryos from blastocyst to early somite stage. Dev. Biol., 68: 453-461.

HSU, Y.C. (1980) Embryo growth and differentiation factors in embryonic sera of mammals. Dev. Biol., 76: 465-474.

HSU, Y.C. (1981) Regulation of mouse embryogenesis by exogenous growth factors. In: Neubert, D. & Merker, H.-J., ed. Culture techniques. Applicability for studies on prenatal differentiation and toxicity, Berlin, New York, Walter de Gruyter Publ., pp. 83-96.

HUGHES, E.W. & PALMER, A.K. (1980) An assessment of pre-weaning development and behaviour in safety evaluation studies, Annual Meeting of the ETS, Münster.

HURLEY, L.S. & SHRADER, R.E. (1972) Congenital malformations of the nervous system in zinc deficient rats. In: Pfeiffer, C.C., ed. Neurobiology of the trace metals zinc and copper. pp. 7-51 (Int. Rev. Neurol., Suppl., 1).

IARC (1980) Long-term and short-term screening assays for carcinogens: a critical appraisal, Lyons, International Agency for Research on Cancer (IARC Monographs on the evaluation of the carcinogenic risk of chemicals to humans, Suppl. 2).

IARC (1982) Chemicals, industrial processes, and industries associated wih cancer in humans, Lyons, International Agency for Research on Cancer (IARC Monographs on the evaluation of the carcinogenic risk of chemicals to humans, Suppl. 4).

ILLSLEY, N.P. & LAMARTINIERE, C.A. (1979) Prenatal programming of hepatic monoamine oxidase by 5,5-diphenylhydantoin. Biochem. Pharmacol., 28: 2585-2590.

IRLG (1979) Interagency Regulatory Liaison Group, Scientific basis for identification of potential carcinogens and risk estimation. J. Natl Cancer Inst., 63: 243-268.

IVANKOVIC, S. (1979) Teratogenic and carcinogenic effects of some chemicals during prenatal life in rats, Syrian golden hamsters, and minipigs. In: Perinatal carcinogenesis. Natl Cancer Inst. Monogr., 51: 103-115.

IVANKOVIC, S. & DRUCKREY, H. (1968) [Transplacental induction of malignant tumours of the nervous system. I. Ethylnitroso urea with BD IX-rats.] Z. Krebsforsch, 71: 320-360 (in German).

JACOBSON, M. (1978) Developmental neurobiology, New York, Plenum Press.

JELINEK, R. (1979) Embryotoxicity assay on morphogenetic systems. In: Benešova, O., Rychter, Z., & Jelinek, R., ed. Evaluation of embryotoxicity, mutagenicity and carcinogenicity risks in new drugs, Prague, Univerzita Karlova, pp. 195-205.

JELINEK, R. & PETERKA, M. (1981) Morphogenetic systems and in vitro techniques in teratology. In: Neubert, D. & Merker, H.-J., ed. Culture techniques. Applicability for studies on prenatal differentiation and toxicity. Berlin, New York, Walter de Gruyter Publ., pp. 553-557.

JELINEK, R. & RYCHTER, Z. (1979) Morphogenetic systems and the central phenomena of teratology. In: Persand, T.-V.N., ed. New trends in experimental teratology, Lancaster, MTP Press, pp. 41-67.

JELINEK, R., RYCHTER, Z., & PETERKA, M. (1976) Cs. Authors Certificate No. 191, 501, Praha.

JICK, H., SHIOTA, K., SHEPARD, T.H., HUNTER, J.R., STERGACHIS, A., MADSEN, S., & PORTER, J.B. (1982) Vaginal spermicides and miscarriage seen primarily in the emergency room. Teratog. Carcinog. Mutag., 2: 205-210.

JOHANSON, I.B. & HALL, W.G. (1979) Appetitive learning in 1-day-old rat pups. Science, 205: 419-421.

JOHN, D.M., CLARK, S.M., & CLARK, R. (1982) Temporal shifts in the incidence of skeletal variations in the CD rat. In: Abstracts of the 10th Meeting of the European Teratology Society, Norwich, England.

JOHNSON, E.M. (1980) A subvertebrate system for rapid determination of potential teratogenic hazards. J. environ. Pathol. Toxicol., 4: 153-156.

JOHNSON, E.M. (1981) Screening for teratogenic hazards: Nature of the problems. Ann. Rev. Pharmacol. Toxicol., 21: 417-429.

JOHNSON, E.M., GORMAN, R.M., GABEL, B.E.G., & GEORGE, M.E. (1982) The hydra attentuata system for detection of teratogenic hazards. Teratog. Carcinog. Mutag. (in press).

JOHNSTON, M.C. & PRATT, R.M. (1975) A developmental approach to teratology. In: Berry, C.L. & Poswillo, D.E., ed. Teratology, trends and applications, New York, Springer-Verlag, pp. 2-16.

JONES, B.J. & ROBERTS, D.J. (1968) The quantitative measurement of motor inco-ordination in naive mice using an accelerating rotarod. J. Pharm. Pharmacol., 20: 302-304.

JOSSO, N. (1974) Effect of $PGA_2$ and $PGB_1$ on the rat foetal müllerian duct << in vitro>> absence of relationship to testicular anti-müllerian hormone. Biomedicine, 21: 225-229.

JOST, A. & BERGERARD, Y. (1949) Culture in vitro d'ébauches du tractus génital du foetus de rat. C.R. Soc. Biol., 143: 608-609.

JURGELSKI, W. Jr, HUDSON, P.M., FALK, H.L., & KOTIN, P. (1976) Embryonal neoplasms in the opossum: a new model for solid tumors of infancy and childhood. Science, 193: 328-332.

JUSKO, W.J. (1972) Pharmacodynamic principles in chemical teratology: dose effect relationships. J. Pharmacol. exp. Therap., 183: 469-480.

KALLAI, L. (1967) Pharmaco-ecology and some nutritional paradoxes. In: M.L. Conalty, ed. Husbandry of laboratory animals, London, Academic Press.

KALOJANOVA, F. (1982) Evaluation of pesticide toxicity for sanitary registration. In: Toxicology of pesticides, Proceedings of a seminar, Sofia, Bulgaria, 31 August-12 September, 1981. Interim document 9, pp. 265-274.

KALTER, H. (1965) Interplay of intrinsic and extrinsic factors. In: Wilson, J.G. & Warkany, J., ed. Teratology Principals & Techniques, Chicago, University of Chicago Press, 279 pp.

KALTER, H. & WARKANY, J. (1983) Congenital malformations. Etiology factors and their role in prevention. Part I & II. New Engl. J. Med., 308: 424-431, 491-497.

KARKINEN-JÄÄSKELÄINEN, M., SAXEN, L., VAHERI, A., & LEINIKKI, P. (1975) Rubella cataract _in vitro_: sensitive period of the developing human lens. _J. exp. Med._, _141_: 1238-1248.

KAUFFMAN, S.L. (1976) Susceptibility of fetal lung to transplacental 1-ethyl-1-nitrosourea: its relation to epithelial proliferation. _J. Natl Cancer Inst._, _57_: 821-825.

KAVLOCK, R.J., MEYER, E., & GRABOWSKI, C.T. (1980) Studies on the developmental toxicity to ozone: postnatal effects. _Toxicol. Lett._, _5_: 3-9.

KERLEY, M.A. & KOLLAR, E.J. (1978) _In vitro_ inhibition of mouse dental development by tetracycline. _J. exp. Zool._, _203_: 89-98.

KHERA, K.S. (1976) Significance of metabolic patterns in teratogenic testing for food safety. _Clin. Toxicol._, _9_: 773-790.

KHERA, K.S. (1981) Common fetal aberrations and their teratologic significance: a review. _Fundam. appl. Toxicol._, _1_: 13-18.

KHERA, K.S. (1983) Materno-fetal toxicity - a possible cause of fetal malformations in the mouse. _Teratology_, _27_: 56A-57A.

KHERA, K.S. (in press) Adverse effects in humans and animals of prenatal exposure to selected therapeutic drugs and estimation of embryo-fetal sensitivity of animals for human risk assessment: a review. _Issues and Reviews in Teratology_, _2_.

KHERA, K.S. & RUDDICK, J.A. (1973) Polychlorodibenzo-_p_-dioxins: perinatal effects and the dominant lethal test in Wistar rats. In: Blaire, E.H., ed. _Chlorodioxins: origin and fate_. _Adv. Chem. Ser._, _120_: 70-85.

KIMMEL, C.A. (1976) Behavioural teratology: overview. _Environ. Health Perspect._, _18_: 73.

KIMMEL, C.A. & BUELKE-SAM, J., ed. (1981) _Developmental toxicology_, New York, Raven Press.

KIMMEL, C.A., MOORE, W. Jr, HYSELL, D.K., & STARA, J.F. (1974) Teratogenicity of hexachlorophene in rats. _Arch. environ. Health_, _28_: 43-48.

KIMMEL, G.L., SMITH, K., KOCHHAR, D.M., & PRATT, R.M. (1982) Overview of _in vitro_ teratogenicity testing; aspects of validation and application to screening. _Teratog. Carcinog. Mutag._, _2_: 221-229.

KLEE-TRIESCHMANN, U. & NEUBERT, D. (1981) Preliminary communication on the feasibility of culturing whole embryos in a chemically defined medium. In: Neubert, D. & Merker, H.-J., ed. _Culture techniques. Applicability for studies on prenatal differentiation and toxicity_, Berlin, New York, Walter de Gruyter Publ., pp. 97-100.

KLEIHUES, P., DOERJER, G., SWENBERG, J.A., HAUENSTEIN, E., BÜCHELER, J., & COOPER, H.K. (1979a) DNA repair as regulatory factor in the organotropy of alkylating carcinogens. _Arch. Toxicol., Suppl._, _2_: 253-261.

KLEIHUES, P., COOPER, H.K., BUECHELER, J., KOLAR, G.F., & DIESSNER, H. (1979b) Mechanism of perinatal tumour induction by neurooncogenic alkylnitrosoureas and dialkylarytriazenes. Perinatal Carcinogenesis, _NCI Monograph_, _51_: 227.

KLEIN, N.W., PLENEFISCH, J.D., CAREY, S.W., CHATOT, C.L., & CLAPPER, M.L. (1981) Evaluation of serum teratogenic activity using rat embryo cultures. In: Neubert, D. & Merker, H.-J., ed. _Culture techniques. Applicability for studies on prenatal differentiation and toxicity_, Berlin, New York, Walter de Gruyter Publ., pp. 67-81.

KLEIN, N.W., VOGLER, M.A., CHATOT, C.L., & PIERRO, L.J. (1980) The use of cultured rat embryos to evaluate the teratogenic activity of serum: cadmium and cyclophosphamide. _Teratology_, _21_: 199-208.

KOCH, W. (1974) The effects of azetidine-2-carboxylic acid on cultured incisors of embryonic mice. _Anat. Rec._, _178_: 393-394.

KOCHHAR, D.M. (1970) Effect of azetidine-2-carboxylic acid, a proline analog, on chondrogenesis in cultured limb buds. In: Bass, R., Beck, F., Merker, H.-J., Neubert, D., & Randhahn, B., ed. _Metabolic pathways in mammalian embryos during organogenesis and its modification by drugs_, Berlin, Free University Press, pp. 475-482.

KOCHHAR, D.M. (1975a) The use of _in vitro_ procedures in teratology. _Teratology_, _11_: 273-288.

KOCHHAR, D.M. (1975b) Assessment of teratogenic response in cultured postimplantation mouse embryos: effects of hydroxyurea. In: Neubert, D. & Merker, H.-J., ed. New approaches to the evaluation of abnormal embryonic development, Stuttgart, Georg Thieme Publ., pp. 250-277.

KOCHHAR, D.M. (1976) Elucidation of mechanisms underlying experimental mammalian teratogenesis through a combination of whole embryo, organ culture, and cell culture methods. In: Ebert, J.D. & Marois, M., ed. Tests of teratogenicity in vitro, Amsterdam, North-Holland Publ., pp. 485-494.

KOLESNICENKO, T.S., POPOVA, N.V., & ŠABAD, L. M. (1978) [Liver tumours in mice induced by prenatal and postnatal exposure to orthoaminoasotoluene.] Bull. exp. Biol., 2: 193-202 (in Russian).

KOLLAR, E.J. (1973) Effect of α,α-dipyridyl on organ cultures of embryonic mouse tooth germs. J. dent. Res., 52: 145.

KOROLEV, A.A. & AGAREVA, E.N. (1983) [Sanitary and toxicological assessment of certain asodyes and their transformation products.] Hig. i. Sanit., 1: 15-18 (in Russian).

KREMERS, P., GOUJON, F., DE GRAEVE, J., VAN CANTFORT, J., & GIELEN, J.E. (1981) Multiplicity of cytochrome P-450 in primary fetal hepatocytes in culture. Eur. J. Biochem., 116: 67-72.

KREWSKI, D. & VAN RYZIN, J. (1981) Dose response models for quantal response toxicity data. In: Scorgo, M., Dawson, D., Rao, J.N.K., & Salch, E., ed. Statistics and related topics, New York, North-Holland, pp. 201-231.

KROWKE, R. & NEUBERT, D. (1977) Embryonic intermediary metabolism under normal and pathological conditions. In: Wilson, J.G. & Fraser, F.C., ed. Handbook of Teratology, New York, London, Plenum Press, Vol. II, pp. 117-151.

KUČERA, J. (1961a) [Registration of congenital malformations in the CSR.] Prakt. Lek. (Praha), 41: 487-490 (in Czech).

KUČERA, J. (1961b) The frequency of congenital malformations in the CSR, and factors influencing it. I. Cas. Lek. Ces., 100: 1609-1614.

KUČERA, J. (1968a) [Syndrome of caudal regression and its significance in the study of etiology and/or prevention of congenital malformations.] Cs. Pediat., 23: 17-25 (in Czech).

KUČERA, J. (1968b) Exposure to fat solvents: a possible cause of sacral agenesis in man, J. Pediat., 72: 857-859.

KUČERA, J. (1971a) Movement of the frequencies of congenital malformations in time and space. Soc. Biol., 18: 422-430.

KUČERA, J. (1971b) Patterns of congenital anomalies in the offspring of women exposed to different drugs and/or chemicals during pregnancy. Teratology, 4: 492.

KUČERA, J. (1977) Relation between population genetics and population teratology. In: Szabo, L. & Papp. S., ed. Proceedings of Medical Genetics, Budapest, Amsterdam, Akad. Kiado, pp. 449-473.

KURILO, L.F., LEONOV, B.V., IGNATJEVA, E.L., SKIRTLADZE, Z.Š., & HILKEVIČ, L.H. (1982) [Some morpho-functional data about the follicular system of the human ovary.] In: [Current aspects of studies of women's reproductive functions.] Moscow, pp. 41-46 (in Russian).

KURILO, L.F., LEONOV, B.V., IGNATJEVA, E.L., SEKERTLADZE, Z.Š., & HIULKEVIČ, L.B. (in press) [Oxitetracillinum and 17-B-estradiol inhibition of oogonia proliferation in human fetal ovary in culture.] Obstetrics and Gynaecology (in Russian).

KVITNIZKAJA, V.A. & KOLENSNIČENKO, T.S. (1971) [About transplacental blastomogenic action zineb on mice offspring.] Vop. Onkol., 1: 49-50 (in Russian).

KWASIGROCH, T.E., SKALKO, R.G., & CHURCH, J.K. (1981) Development of limb buds in organ culture: examination of hydroxyurea enhancement of bromodeoxyuridine toxicity using image analysis. In: Neubert, D. & Merker, H.-J., ed. Culture techniques. Applicability for studies on prenatal differentiation and toxicity, Berlin, New York, Walter de Gruyter Publ., pp. 237-253.

LAHTI, A. & SAXEN, L. (1967) Effect of hydrocortisone on the closure of palatal shelves in vivo and in vitro. Nature (Lond.), 216: 1217-1218.

LAMBSON, R.O. (1966) An electron microscopic visualization of transport across rat visceral yolk sac. Am. J. Anat., 118: 21-52.

LANGMAN, J. (1969) Medical embryology, 2nd edition, Baltimore, Williams and Wilkins.

LANGMAN, J., WEBSTER, W., & RODIER, P. (1975) Morphological and behavioural abnormalities caused by insults to the CNS in the perinatal period. In: Berry, C.L. & Poswillo, D.E., ed. Teratology, trends and applications, New York, Springer-Verlag, pp. 182-200.

LAPOINTE, G. & NOSAL, G. (1979) A rat model of neurobehavioral development. Experientia, Basel, 35: 205-207.

LAQUEUR, G.L. & SPATZ, M. (1973) Transplacental induction of tumours and malformations in rats with cycasin and methylazoxymethanol. In: Tomatis, L., Mohr, U., & Davis, W., ed. Transplacental carcinogenesis, Lyons, International Agency for Research on Cancer, pp. 59-64 (IARC Scientific Publications No. 4).

LAROCHE, M.J. (1965) Influence of environment on drug activity in laboratory animals. Food Cosmet. Toxicol., 3: 177-191.

LASNITZKI, I. & MIZUNO, T. (1981) Interaction of epithelium and mesenchyme in the induction of foetal rat and mouse prostate glands by androgens in organ culture. In: Neubert, D. & Merker, H.-J., ed. Culture techniques. Applicability for studies on prenatal differentiation and toxicity, Berlin, New York, Walter de Gruyter Publ., pp. 359-369.

LEBLOND, C.P. & CLERMONT (1952) Definition of the stages of the cycle of the seminiferous epithelium in the rat. Ann. NY Acad. Sci., 55: 548-573.

LEEMING, N.M., COZENS, D.D., & PALMER, A.K. (1982) Points for consideration in the design of multigeneration studies. In: Abstracts of the 10th Meeting of the European Teratology Society, Norwich.

LEONOV, B.V. (1979) [Sexual hormones and hormone-like substances in early embryogenesis.] Moscow, Medicina, p. 160 (in Russian).

LESSMÖLLMANN, U., NEUBERT, D., & MERKER, H.-J. (1975) Mammalian limb buds differentiating in vitro as a test system

LEBLOND, C.P. & CLERMONT, Y. (1952) Definition of the stages of the cycle of the seminiferous epithelium in the rat. Ann. NY Acad. Sci., 55: 548-573.

LEEMING, N.M., COZENS, D.D., & PALMER, A.K. (1982) Points for consideration in the design of multigeneration studies. In: Abstracts of the 10th Meeting of the European Teratology Society, Norwich.

LEONOV, B.V. (1979) [Sexual hormones and hormone-like substances in early embryogenesis.] Moscow, Medicina, p. 160 (in Russian).

LESSMÖLLMANN, U., NEUBERT, D., & MERKER, H.-J. (1975) Mammalian limb buds differentiating in vitro as a test system for the evaluation of embryotoxic effects. In: Neubert, D. & Merker, H.-J., ed. New approaches to the evaluation of abnormal embryonic development, Stuttgart, Georg Thieme Publ., pp. 99-113.

LESSMÖLLMANN, U., HINZ, N., & NEUBERT, D. (1976) In vitro system for toxicological studies on the development of mammalian limb buds in a chemically defined medium. Arch. Toxicol., 36: 169-176.

LEUNG, T.S. & BULKLEY, R.V. (1979) Effects of petroleum hydrocarbons on length of incubation and hatching success in the Japanese medaka. Bull. environ. Contam. Toxicol., 23: 236-243.

LEVITT, D., HO, P.L., & DORFMAN, A. (1975) Effect of 5-bromodeoxyuridine on ultrastructure of developing limb bud cells in vitro. Dev. Biol., 43: 75-90.

LEWIN, B. (1980) Gene expression, Vol. 2. Eukaryotic chromosome, John Wiley & Sons.

LEWIS, C.A., PRATT, R.M., PENNYPACKER, J.P., & HASSELL, J.R. (1978) Inhibition of limb chondrogenesis in vitro by vitamin A: alterations in cell surface characteristics. Dev. Biol., 64: 31-47.

LEWIS, P.D. & PATEL, A.J. (1980) Psychtropic drugs and brain development: effects on cell acquisition. In: di Benedetta, C., ed. Multidisciplinary approach to brain development, Amsterdam, Elsevier, North Holland, pp. 509-517.

LIDDIARD, C., BRENDEL, K., & NAU, H. (1978) Drug metabolism in cultures of isolated hepatocytes of the human fetus, the newborn pig and the adult rat. In: Neubert, D., Merker, H.-J., Nau, H., Langman, J., ed. Role of pharmacokinetics in prenatal and perinatal toxicology, Stuttgart, Georg Thieme Publ., pp. 91-108.

LIKHACHEV, A.J. (1971) [Blastomogenesis induced by the combined transplacental and postnatal exposure to N-nitrosodiethyl-amine (NDEA) in mice]. Vopr. Onkol., 17(4): 64-69 (in Russian).

LIKHACHEV, A.J., ALEXANDROV, V.A., ANISIMOV, V.N., BESPALOV, V.G., KORSAKOV, M.V., OVSJANNIKOV, A.I., POPOVIC, I.G., NAPALKOV, N.P., & TOMATIS, L. (1983) Persistence of methylated purines in the DNA of various rat fetal and maternal tissues and carcinogenesis in the offspring following a single transplacental dose of N-methyl-N-nitrosourea. Int. J. Cancer, 31: 779-784.

LJUNGBERG, T. & UNGERSTEDT, U. (1976) Automatic registration of behaviour related to dopamine and noradrenaline transmission. Eur. J. Pharmacol., 36: 181-188.

LOPATA, A., MARTIN, M., OLIVA, K., & JOHNSTON, I. (1982) Embryonic development and blastocyst implantation following in vitro fertilization and embryo transfer. Fertil. Steril., 38: 682-687.

LUCIER, G.W. & MCDANIEL, O.S. (1979) Developmental toxicology of the halogenated aromatics: Effects on enzyme development. Ann. NY Acad. Sci., 77: 449-457.

LUCIER, G.W., SONAWANE, B.R., MCDANIEL, O.S., & HOOK, G.E.R. (1975) Postnatal stimulation of hepatic microsomal enzymes following administration of TCDD to pregnant rats. Chem. Biol. Interact., 11: 15-26.

LUNDBORG, P. & ENGEL, J. (1978) Neurochemical brain changes associated with behavioural disturbances after early treatment with psychotropic drugs. In: Vernadakis, ed. Maturation of neurotransmission, Basel, S. Karger, pp. 226-235.

LÜSCHER, M. (1946) [Inhibition of regeneration of the tail of xenopus larvae by colchicine and analysis of its action during development.] Helv. Physiol. Pharmacol. Acta, 4: 465 (in German).

LÜSCHER, M. (1955) [The regeneration in Zoology.] In: Handbuch der allgemeinen Pathologie, Berlin, Springer-Verlag, Vol. 6, Part I, pp. 406-440 (in German).

LUTWAK-MANN, C. (1973) Drugs and the blastocyst. In: Boréus, L.O., ed. Fetal pharmacology, New York, Raven Press Publ., pp. 419-442.

MACKENZIE, K.M., LUCIER, G.W., & MCLACHLAN, J.A. (1979a) Infertility in mice exposed prenatally to benzo-[α]-pyrene. (BP) Teratology, 19: 37A.

MACKENZIE, K.M., LUCIER, G.W., & MCLACHLAN, J.A. (1979b) Infertility in mice following prenatal exposure to 9,10-dimethyl-1,2-benzanthracene (DMBA). In: Proceedings of the 12th Annual Meeting of the Society for the Study of Reproduction, Quebec, p. 30A.

MAEKAWA, A. & ODASHIMA, S. (1975) Induction of tumours of the nervous system in the ACI/N rat with 1-butyl-1-nitrosourea administered transplacentally, neonatally, or via maternal milk. Gann. Jpn. J. Cancer Res., 66(2): 175-183.

MAEKAWA, A., ISHIWATA, H., & ODASHIMA, S. (1977) Transplacental carcinogenesis and chemical determination of 1-butyl-1-nitrosourea in stomach content after simultaneous oral administration of 1-butylurea and sodium nitrite to ACI/N rats. Gann. Jpn. J. Cancer Res., 68(1): 81-87.

MAEKAWA, A., ONODERA, H., FURUTA, K., & ODASHIMA, S. (1980) Transplacental and neonatal carcinogenesis by 1-butyl-1-nitrosourethan in the ACI/N rat. Gann. Jpn. J. Cancer Res., 71: 811-815.

MANTEL, N. & BRYAN, W.R. (1961) "Safety"-testing of carcinogenic agents. J. Natl Cancer Inst., 27: 455-470.

MANTEL, N. & SCHNEIDERMAN, M.A. (1975) Estimating "safe" levels, a hazardous undertaking. Cancer Res., 35: 1379-1386.

MARSDEN, C.A. (1979) The use of doppler shift radar to monitor physiological and drug induced activity patterns in the rat. Pharmacol. Biochem. Behav., 10: 631-635.

MARTIN, G.R. (1978) Advantages and limitations of teratocarcinoma stem cells as models of development. In: Hohnsonn, M.M., ed. Development in mammals, Elsevier, North Holland, Biomedical Press, Amsterdam, pp. 225-261.

MARTINOVITCH, P.N. (1938) The development in vitro of the mammalian gonad. Ovary and ovogenesis. Proc. Roy. Soc. Lond., 125: 232-249.

MATEYKO, J.M. (1967) Developmental modification in Arbacia punctulate by various metabolic substances. Biol. Bull., 13(1): 184-228.

MATSUMOTO, N. & SPINDLE, A. (1982) Sensitivity of early mouse embryos to methylmercury toxicity. Toxicol. appl. Pharmacol., 64: 108-117.

MAUER, R.R., HAFEZ, E.S.E., EHLERS, M.H., & KING, J.R. (1968) Culture of two cell rabbit eggs in chemically defined media. Exp. Cell Res., 52: 293-300.

MCLACHLAN, J.A. & DIXON, R.L. (1973) Reduced fertility in female mice exposed prenatally to procarbazine. Fed. Proc., 32: 2982.

MCLACHLAN, J.A., NEWBOLD, R.R., & BULLOCK, B. (1975) Reproductive tract lesions in male mice exposed prenatally to diethylstilbestrol. Science, 190: 991-992.

MCLACHLAN, J.A., NEWBOLD, R.R., KORACH, K.S., LAMB, J.C., & SUZUKI, Y. (1981) Transplacental toxicology: prenatal factors influencing postnatal fetility. In: Kimmel, C.A. & Buelke-Sam, J., ed. Developmental Toxicology, New York, Raven Press, pp. 213-232.

MCLAREN, A. & BIGGERS, J.D. (1958) Successful development and birth of mice cultivated in vitro as early embryos. Nature (Lond.): 182: 877.

MELBERG, P.E., AHLENIUS, S., ENGEL, J., & LUNDBORG, P. (1976) Ontogenetic development of locomotor activity and rate of tyrosine hydroxylation. Psychopharmacology, 49: 119-123.

MELLO, N.K. (1975) Behavioral toxicology: a developing discipline. Fed. Proc., 34: 1832-1834.

MERKER, H.-J. (1975) Significance of the limb bud culture system for investigations of teratogenic mechanisms. In: Neubert, D. & Merker, H.-J., ed. New approaches to the evaluation of abnormal embryonic development, Stuttgart, Georg Thieme Publ., pp. 161-199.

MERKER, H.-J. & GÜNTHER, TH. (1979) The influence of insulin, cAMP and the calcium ionophore X 537 A on the growth of the cartilage anlagen of limb buds in vitro. Experientia, Basel: 35: 1307-1308.

MERKER, H.-J., LILJA, S., & GUNTHER, TH. (1978a) Formation of an atypical collagen and cartilage pattern in limb bud cultures by highly sulfated GAG. _Virchow's Arch._, _380_: 11-30.

MERKER, H.-J., GÜNTHER, TH., & KRÜGER, U. (1978b) Effect of 4-methylumbelliferyl-φ-D-xylopyranoside on the morphology of embryonic cartilage in limb bud cultures. _Teratology_, _18_: 291-310.

MERKER, H.-J., ZIMMERMANN, B., BARRACH, H.-J., GRUNDMANN, K., & EBEL, H. (1980a) Simulation of steps of limb skeletogenesis _in vitro_. In: Merker, H.-J., Nau, H., & Neubert, D., ed. _Teratology of the limbs_, Berlin, Walter de Gruyter Publ., pp. 137-151.

MERKER, H.-J., ZIMMERMANN, B., & GRUNDMANN, K. (1980b) Differentiation of isolated blastemal cells from limb buds into chondroblasts. In: Richards, R.J. & Rajan, K.T., ed. _Tissue culture in medical research (II)_, Oxford, New York, Pergamon Press, pp. 31-39.

MERKER, H.-J., ZIMMERMANN, B., & RISO, J. (1981) The embryonic lung as _in vitro_ model for testing teratogenic substances. In: Neubert, D. & Merker, H.-J., ed. _Culture techniques. Applicability for studies on prenatal differentiation and toxicity_, Berlin, New York, Walter de Gruyter Publ., pp. 301-317.

MERKURJEWA, R.W., RACHMANIN, Y.A., BURMANTOWA, N.P., JANKELEWITSCH, I.B., & DOLINSKAYA, S.I. (1983) [The influence of orally administered formaldehyde on embryogenesis and enzyme activity.] _Z. Ges. Hyg._, _29_(2): 66-68 (in German).

MICHAELSON, I.A., GREENLAND, R.D., & SAUERHOFF, M.W. (1974) Studies of lead encephalopathy in the developing rat. In: _Proceedings of the CEC-EPA-WHO International Symposium - Recent advances in the assessment of the health effects of environmental pollution, Vol. II, Paris, June_, CEC Directorate General, Scientific and Technical Information and Information Management.

MILLER, J.F., WILLIAMSON, E., GLUE, J., GORDON, Y.B., GRUDZINSKAS, J.G., & SYKES, A. (1980) Fetal loss after implantation. A prospective study. _Lancet_, _I_: 554-556.

MILLER, R.W. (1977) Relationship between human teratogens and carcinogens. _J. Natl Cancer Inst._, _58_: 471-474.

MILUNSKY, A., GRAEF, J.W., & GAYNOR, M.F. (1968) Methotrexate-induced congenital malformations. J. Pediatr., 72: 790-795.

MIRKIN, B.L. & SINGH, S. (1976) Placental transfer of pharmacologically active molecules. In: Mirkin, B.L., ed. Perinatal pharmacology and therapeutics, New York, Academic Press, pp. 1-69.

MISANIN, J.R., NAGY, Z.M., KEISER, E.F., & BOWEN, W. (1971) Emergence of long-term memory in the neonatal rat. J. comp. Physiol. Psychol., 77: 188-199.

MITCHELL, C.L. (1978) Target organ toxicity: nervous system. Environ. Health Perspect., 26: 3-4.

MOHR, U., REZNIK-SCHÜLLER, H., REZNIK, G., & HILFRICH, J. (1975) Transplacental effects of diethylnitrosamine in Syrian hamsters as related to different days of administration during pregnancy. J. Natl Cancer Inst., 55: 681-683.

MOSCONA, A. & MOSCONA, H. (1952) The dissociation and aggregation of cells from organ rudiments of the early chick embryo. J. Anat., 86: 287-301.

MURPHY, M.L. (1965) Factors influencing teratogenic response to drugs. In: Wilson, J.G. & Warkany, J., ed. Teratology, Chicago, London, The University of Chicago Press, pp. 145-184.

NAPALKOV, N.P. (1973) Some general considerations on the problem of transplacental carcinogenesis. In: Tomatis, L., Mohr, U., & Davis, W., ed. Transplacental carcinogenesis, Lyons, International Agency for Research on Cancer, pp. 1-13 (IARC Scientific Publications No. 4).

NAPALKOV, N.P. & ALEXANDROV, V.A. (1968) On the effects of blastomogenic substances on the organism during embryogenesis. Z. Krebsforsch., 71: 32-50.

NAPALKOV, N.P. & ANISIMOV, V.N. (1979) Transplacental effect of diethylstilbestrol in female rats. Cancer Lett., 6: 107-114.

NAS (1977) Principles and procedures for evaluating the toxicology of household substances. 7. Reproduction and teratogenicity tests, Washington, DC, US National Academy of Sciences, pp. 99-110.

NAS (1977) National Academy of Sciences, Drinking water and health, Washington, DC, Printing and Publishing Office, National Academy of Sciences, pp. 24-54 (prepared for the US Environmental Protection Agency under contract no. 68-01-3139).

NAS (1983) National Academy of Sciences, Committee on the institutional means or assessment of risk to public health, commission on life sciences, National Research Council, Risk assessment in the Federal Government: Managing the process, Washington, DC, National Academy Press, ISBN D-309-03349-7.

NAU, H., LIDDIARD, C., BRENDEL, K., WITTFOHT, W., & LANGE, J. (1977) Benzodiazepine metabolism studies in organ and isolated cell cultures of human fetal liver by a gas chromatography mass spectrometer computer system. In: Eggstein, M. & Liebich, H.M., ed. Mass spectrometry and combined techniques in medicine, clinical chemistry and clinical biochemistry, Tübingen University Press, pp. 346-358.

NAU, H., ZIERER, R., SPIELMAN, H., NEUBERT, D., & GANSAU, CH. (1981) A new model for embryotoxicity testing: teratogenicity and pharmacokinetics of valproic acid following constant-rate administration in the mouse using human therapeutic drug and metabolite concentrations. Life Sci., 29: 2803-2814.

NEUBERT, D. (1980a) [Extrapolations from animal studies. Prospective in vitro models as substitute for long-term tests.] In: Schnieders, B. & Grosdanoff, P., ed. Zur Problematik von chronischen Toxizitätsprüfungen, AMI-Berichte 1/1980, Berlin, Dietrich Reimer Verlag, pp. 277-287 (in German).

NEUBERT, D. (1980b) Teratogenicity: any relationship to carcinogenicity? In: Montesano, R., Bartsch, H., Tomatis, L., & Davis, W., ed. Molecular and cellular aspects of carcinogen screening tests, Lyons, International Agency for Research on Cancer, pp. 169-178 (IARC Scientific Publications No. 27).

NEUBERT, D. (1982) The use of culture techniques in studies on prenatal toxicity. Pharmac. Ther., 18: 397-434.

NEUBERT, D. (1983) [Can mutagenicity tests or other in vitro methods replace carcinogenicity or other long-term in vivo studies?] In: Grosdanoff, P., Schneiders, B., & Überla, K., ed. Arzneimittel Sicherheit, MMV, bga Berichte 1/1983, pp. 83-88 (in German).

NEUBERT, D. & BARRACH, H.J. (1977b) Techniques applicable to study morphogenetic differentiation of limb buds in organ culture. In: Neubert, D., Merker, H.-J., & Kwasigroch, T.E., ed. _Methods in prenatal toxicology. Evaluation of embryotoxic effects in experimental animals_, Stuttgart, Georg Thieme Publ., pp. 241-251.

NEUBERT, D. & BLUTH, U. (1981a) Feasibility of storing embryonic tissues for subsequent use in organ culture. In: Neubert, D. & Merker, H.-J., ed. _Culture techniques. Applicability for studies on prenatal differentiation and toxicity_, Berlin, New York, Walter de Gruyter Publ., pp. 171-173.

NEUBERT, D. & BLUTH, U. (1981b) Limb bud organ cultures from mouse embryos after apparent induction of monooxygenases _in utero_. Effects of cyclophosphamide,, dimethylnitrosamine and some thalidomide derivatives. In: Neubert, D. & Merker, H.-J., ed. _Culture techniques. Applicability for studies on prenatal differentiation and toxicity_, Berlin, New York, Walter de Gruyter Publ., pp. 175-195.

NEUBERT, D. & CHAHOUD, I. (in press) Significance of species differences in pre- and perinatal toxicity. _Z. Histochem._

NEUBERT, D. & DILLMANN, I. (1972) Embryotoxic effects in mice treated with 2,4,5-trichlorophenoxyacetic acid and 2,3,7,8-tetrachlorodibenzo-p-dioxin. _Naunyn-Schmiedebergs Arch. Pharmacol._, _272_: 243-264.

NEUBERT, D. & MERKER, H.-J., ed. (1981) _Culture techniques. Applicability for studies on prenatal differentiation and toxicity_, Berlin, New York, Walter de Gruyter Publ., pp. 1-607.

NEUBERT, D. & RAUTENBERG, M. (1976) Activity of nuclear DNA-dependent RNA polymerases in mouse limb buds differentiating _in vivo_ or in organ culture. _Hoppe-Seyler's Z. Physiol. Chem._, _357_: 1623-1635.

NEUBERT, D., PETERS, H., TESKE, S., KÖHLER, E., & BARRACH, H.-J. (1971) Studies on the problem of "aerobic glycolysis" occuring in mammalian embryos. _Naunyn-Schmiedebergs Arch. Pharmak_, _268_: 235-241.

NEUBERT, D., ZENS, P., ROTHENWALLNER, A., & MERKER, H.-J. (1973) A survey of the embryotoxic effects of TCDD in mammalian species. _Environ. Health Perspect._, _5_: 67-79.

NEUBERT, D., MERKER, H.-J., & TAPKEN, S. (1974) Comparative studies on the prenatal development of mouse extremities _in_ vivo and in organ culture. Naunyn-Schmiedeberg's Arch. Pharmacol., 286: 251-270.

NEUBERT, D., MERKER, H.-J., BARRACH, H.-J., & LESSMÖLLMANN, U. (1976) Biochemical and teratological aspects of mammalian limb bud development in vitro. In: Ebert, J.D. & Marois, M., ed. Tests of teratogenicity in vitro, Amsterdam, New York, Oxford, North-Holland Publ. Comp., pp. 335-365.

NEUBERT, D., LESSMÖLLMANN, U., HINZ, N., DILLMANN, I., & FUCHS, G. (1977a) Interference of 6-mercaptopurine riboside, 6-methylmercaptopurine riboside and azathioprine with the morphogenetic differentiation of mouse extremities in vivo and in organ culture. Naunyn-Schmiedeberg's Arch. Pharmacol., 298: 93-105.

NEUBERT, D., MERKER, H.-J., & KWASIGROCH, T.E., ed. (1977b) Methods in prenatal toxicology, Stuttgart, Georg Thieme Publ.

NEUBERT, D., MERKER, H.-J., NAU, H., & LANGMAN, J., ed. (1978a) Role of pharmacokinetics in prenatal and perinatal toxicology, Stuttgart, Georg Thieme Publ.

NEUBERT, D., TAPKEN, S., & BAUMANN, I. (1978b) Influence of potential thalidomide metabolites and hydrolysis products on limb development in organ culture and on the activity of proline hydroxylase. Further data on our hypothesis on the thalidomide embryopathy. In: Neubert, D., Merker, H.-J., Nau, H., & Langman, J., ed. Role of pharmacokinetics in prenatal and perinatal toxicology, Stuttgart, Georg Thieme Publ., pp. 359-382.

NEUBERT, D., BARRACH, H.J., & MERKER, H.-J. (1980) Drug-induced damage to the embryo or fetus. In: Grundmann, E., ed. Current topics in pathology, Berlin, Heidelberg, New York, Springer-Verlag, pp. 242-324.

NEUKOMM, S. (1969) Action of a carcinogenic tar on the regeneration of the tail of the crested newt. A new possible test for evaluation of substances with teratogenic action. In: Bertelli, A. & Donati, L., ed. Teratology, Amsterdam, Excerpta Medica Found. pp. 11-22.

NEW, D.A.T. (1955) A new technique for the cultivation of the chick embryo in vitro. J. Embryol. exp. Morphol., 3: 326-331.

NEW, D.A.T. (1966a) Development of rat embryos cultured in blood sera. J. Reprod. Fertil., 12: 509-524.

NEW, D.A.T. (1966b) The culture of vertebrate embryos, London, New York, Logos Press - Academic Press, pp. 1-245.

NEW, D.A.T. (1976) Techniques for assessment of teratologic effects: embryo culture. Environ. Health Perspect., 18: 105-110.

NEW, D.A.T. (1978) Whole embryo culture and the study of mammalian embryos during organogenesis. Biol. Rev., 53: 81-122.

NEW, D.A.T., COPPOLA, P.T., & TERRY, S. (1973) Culture of explanted rat embryos in rotating tubes. J. Reprod. Fertil., 35: 135-138.

NEW, D.A.T., COPPOLA, P.T., & COCKROFT, D.L. (1976a) Comparison of growth in vitro and in vivo of post-implantation rat embryos. J. Embryol. exp. Morphol., 36: 133-144.

NEW, D.A.T., COPPOLA, P.T., & COCKROFT, D.L. (1976b) Improved development of head-fold rat embryos in culture resulting from low oxygen and modifications of the culture serum. J. Reprod. Fertil., 48: 219-222.

NICOLOV, I.G. & CHERNOZEMSKY, I.N. (1979) Tumours and hyperplastic lesions in Syrian hamsters following transplacental and neonatal treatment with cigarette smoke condensate. J. Cancer Res. clin. Oncol., 94: 249-256.

NISHIMURA, H. (1971) Incidence of malformations in abortions. In: Fraser, F.C. & McKusick, V.A., ed. Congenital malformations. Proceedings of the Third International Congress, Amsterdam, Princeton, Exerpta Medica, pp. 275-283.

NOMURA, T. (1974) An analysis of the changing urethan response of the developing mouse embryo in relation to mortality, malformation, and neoplasm. Cancer Res., 34: 2217-2231.

NOMURA, T. (1982) Parental exposure to X rays and chemicals induces heritable tumours and anomalies in mice. Nature (Lond.), 296: 575-577.

NORTON, S., MULLENIX, P., & CULVER, B. (1976) Comparison of the structure of hyperactive behaviour in rats after brain damage from X-irradiation, carbon monoxide and pallidal lesions. Brain Res., 116: 49-67.

OAKBERG, E.F. (1956) Duration of spermatogenesis in the mouse and timing of stages of the cycle of the seminiferous epithelium. Amer. J. Anat., 99: 507-516.

OECD (1981) Teratogenicity, Paris, Organization for Economic Co-operation and Development (OECD guidelines for testing of chemicals No. 414).

ONUMA, H., MAURER, R.R., & FOOTE, R.H. (1968) In vitro culture of rabbit ova from early cleavage stages to the blastocyst stage. J. Reprod. Fertil., 16: 491-493.

PAGE, E.W., VILLEE, C.A., & VILLEE, D.B. (1981) Human Reproduction, London, Saunders.

PALMER, A.K. (1967) The relationship between screening tests for drug safety and other teratological investigations. In: Proceedings of a Symposium organized by the Italian Society of Experimental Teratology, Como, Italy (Excerpta Medica International Congress Series No. 173, Teratology).

PALMER, A.K. (1969) The concept of the uniform animal relative to teratogenicity. Carworth Europe Collected Papers, 3: 101-113.

PALMER, A.K. (1974) Statistical analysis and choice of sample units. Teratology, 10: 301-302.

PALMER, A.K. (1976) Assessment of current test procedures. Environ. Health Persp., 18: 97-104.

PALMER, A.K. (1977a) Reproductive toxicology studies and their evaluation. In: Ballantyne, B., ed. Current approaches in toxicology, Bristol, Publ. J. Wright, pp. 54-67.

PALMER, A.K. (1977b) Incidence of sporadic malformations, anomalies and variations in random bred laboratory animals. In: Neubert, D., Merker, H.-J., & Kwasigroch, T.E., ed. Methods in prenatal toxicology, Stuttgart, Georg Thieme Publ., pp. 52-71.

PALMER, A.K. (1978) The design of subprimate animal studies. In: Wilson, J.G. & Fraser, F.C., ed. Handbook of teratology, New York, London, Plenum Press, Vol. 4, pp. 215-253.

PALMER, A.K. (1981) Regulatory requirements for reproductive toxicology: theory and practice. In: Kimmel, C.A. & Buelke-

Sam, J., ed. Developmental toxicology, New York, Raven Press, pp. 259-287.

PATEL, A.J., BENDEK, G., BALAZS, R., & LEWIS, P.D. (1977) Effect of reserpine on cell proliferation in the developing rat brain: a biochemical study. Brain Res., 129: 283-297.

PAVLIK, A. & JELINEK, R. (1979) Effect of cycloheximide administered to rats in early postnatal life: correlation of brain changes with behaviour in adulthood. Brain Res., 167: 200-205.

PAVLIK, A. JELINEK, R., & TEISINGER, J. (1980) Short-term inhibition of protein synthesis applied at brain growth spurt: behavioural teratology model. In: Trojan, S. & Stastny, F., ed. Ontogenesis of brain, Prague, Univ. Carol. Prag., Vol. 3, pp. 397-404.

PEDERSEN, R.A. (1981) Benzo[a]pyrene metabolism in early mouse embryos. In: Neubert, D. & Merker, H.-J., ed. Culture techniques. Applicability for studies on prenatal differentiation and toxicity, Berlin, New York, Walter de Gruyter Publ., pp. 447-454.

PELKONEN, O., JOUPPILA, P., & KÄRKI, N.T. (1972) Effect of maternal cigarette smoking on 3,4-benzpyrene and N-methylaniline metabolism in human fetal liver and placenta. Toxicol. appl. Pharmacol., 23: 399-407.

PELLEGRINO, L. & ALTMAN, J. (1979) Effects of differential interference with postnatal cerebellar neurogenesis on motor performance, activity level and maze learning of rats: a development study. J. comp. Physiol. Psychol., 93: 1-33.

PENNYPACKER, J.P., LEWIS, C.A., & HASSELL, J.R. (1978a) Altered proteoglycan metabolism in mouse limb mesenchyme cell cultures treated with vitamin A. Arch. Biochem. Biophys., 186: 351-358.

PENNYPACKER, J.P., WILK, A.L., & MARTIN, G.R. (1978b) In vitro differentiation of mesenchyme cells into chondrocytes: Effect of teratogens in the presence or absence of drug-metabolizing liver preparations. In: Neubert, D., Merker, H.-J., Nau, H., & Langman, J., ed. Role of pharmacokinetics in prenatal and perinatal toxicology, Stuttgart, Georg Thieme Publ., pp. 411-419.

PERRAUD, J. (1976) Levels of spontaneous malformations in the CD rat and CD-1 mouse. Lab. anim. Sci., 26: 293-300.

PHILLIPS, M., ADAMS, J., & BUELKE-SAM, J. (1980) Righting vs. negative geotaxis: a methodological evaluation. Teratology, 21: 60-61A.

PINTO-MACHADO, J. (1970) Influence of prenatal administration of busulfan on the postnatal development of mice. Production of a syndrome including hypoplasia of the thymus. Teratology, 3: 363-370.

PLATZEK, T., BOCHERT, G., SCHNEIDER, W., & NEUBERT, D. (1982) Embryotoxicity induced by alkylating agents: 1. Ethymethanesulfonate as a teratogen in mice. Arch. Toxicol., 51: 1-25.

POPOV, V.B., VAIŠMAN, B.L., & PUCHKOV, V.F. (1981) [Embryotoxic action of cyclophosphamide after biotransformation in vitro on development of rat embryos.] Bull. exp. Biol. Med., 91(5): 613-615 (in Russian, English abstract).

PRATT, R.M. (1983) Mechanisms of chemically-induced cleft palate. Trends pharmacol. Sci., 4: 160-162.

PRATT, R.M., YONEDA, T., SILVER, M.H., & SALOMON, D.S. (1980) Involvement of glucocorticoids and epidermal growth factor in secondary palate development. In: Pratt, R.M. & Christiansen, R.L., ed. Current research trends in prenatal craniofacial development, New York, Amsterdam, Oxford, Elsevier, North-Holland Publ., pp. 235-252.

PRATT, R.M., GROVE, R.I., & WILLIS, W.D. (1982) Prescreening for environmental teratogens using cultured mesenchymal cells from the human embryonic palate. Teratog. Carcinog. Mutag., 2: 313-318.

PRICE, D. & ORTIZ, E. (1965) The role of fetal androgen in sex differentiation in mammals. In: De Haan, R.L. & Ursprung, H., ed. Organogenesis, New York, Rinehart and Winston, pp. 629-652.

QUARLES, J.M. (1981) Transplacental host-mediated assay in the hamster as a rapid screening test for chemical carcinogens. Biol. Res. Pregnancy, 2: 188-194.

RÄIHÄ, N.C.R. & SCHWARTZ, A.L. (1973) Enzyme induction in human fetal liver in organ culture. Enzyme, 15: 330-339.

RAJAN, K.T. (1969) The cultivation in vitro of postfoetal mammalian cartilage and its response to hypervitaminosis A. Exp. Cell Res., 55: 419-423.

RAJAN, K.T. (1974) Human organ culture: applications in the screening of teratogenic drugs. In: Woollam, D.H.M. & Morriss, G.M., ed. Experimental embryology and teratology, London, Elek Science, Vol. 1, pp. 65-89.

RAJAN, K.T., MERKER, H.-J., & WILKINS, M. (1980) Observations on human digits 'in vitro' and its possible role in evaluating teratogens. In: Merker, H.-J., Nau, H., Neubert, D., ed. Teratology of the limbs, Berlin, Walter de Gruyter Publ., pp. 307-324.

RANDALL, P.K. & CAMPBELL, B.A. (1976) Ontogeny of behavioral arousal in rats: effect of maternal and sibling presence. J. comp. Physiol. Psychol., 90: 453-459.

RAUTENBERG, P. & NEUBERT, D. (1975) Methods for the evaluation of mRNA fractions synthesized in limb buds differentiating in organ culture. In: Neubert, D. & Merker, H.-J., ed. New approaches to the evaluation of abnormal embryonic development, Stuttgart, Georg Thieme Publ., pp. 133-144.

REINISCH, J.M. & KAROW, W.G. (1977) Prenatal exposure to synthetic progestins and estrogens: effects on human development. Arch. sex. Behav., 6: 257-288.

REITER, L. (1977) Behavioral toxicology: effects of early postnatal exposure to neurotoxins on development of locomotor activity in the rat. J. occup. Med., 19: 201-204.

REUHL, K.R. & CHANG, L.W. (1979) Effects of methylmercury on the development of the nervous system: a review. Neurotoxicology, 1: 21-55.

REVERBERY, J., ed. (1971) Experimental embryology of marine and fresh-water invertebrates, New York, American Elsevier, p. 570.

RICE, J.M (1969) Transplacental carcinogenesis in mice by 1-ethyl-1-nitrosourea. Ann. NY Acad. Sci., 163: 813-826.

RICE, J.M. (1973a) An overview of transplacental chemical carcinogenesis. Teratology, 8: 113-126.

RICE, J.M. (1973b) The biological behaviour of transplacentally induced tumours in mice. In: Tomatis, L., Mohr, U., & Davis, W., ed. Transplacental carcinogenesis, Lyons, New York, International Agency for Cancer Research, p. 71-83 (IARC Scientific Publications).

RICE, J.M. (1981) Effects of prenatal exposure to chemical carcinogens and methods for their detection. In: Kimmel, C.A. & Buelke-Sam, J., ed. Developmental toxicology, New York, Raven Press, pp. 191-212.

RICE, J.M., LONDON, W.T., PALMER, A.E., SLY, D.L., & WILLIAMS, G.M. (1977) Direct and transplacental carcinogenesis by ethylnitrosourea in the patas monkey (Erythrocebus patas). In: Proceedings of the American Association on Cancer Research., 18 (Mar.): 53.

RISO, J. & ZIMMERMANN, B. (1981) Effects of substances influencing glycosaminoglycan synthesis on lung development in culture. In: Neubert, D. & Merker, H.-J., ed. Culture techniques. Applicability for studies on prenatal differentiation and toxicity, Berlin, New York, Walter de Gruyter Publ., pp. 331-339.

RITTER, E.J. (1977) Altered biosynthesis. In: Wilson, J.G. & Fraser, F.C., ed. Handbook of teratology, Vol. 2, New York, London, Plenum Press, pp. 99-116.

RIVLIN, A.S. & TATOR, C.H. (1977) Objective clinical assessment of motor function after experimental spinal cord injury in the rat. J. Neurosurg., 47: 577-581.

ROBERTS, D.W. & CHAPMAN, J.R. (1981) Concepts essential to the assessment of toxicity to the developing immune system. In: Kimmel, C.A. & Buelke-Sam, J., ed. Developmental toxicology, New York, Raven Press, pp. 167-189.

ROBINSON, E. (1976) The effects of litter size and crowding on position learning by male and female albino rats. Psychol. Res., 26: 61-66.

ROBKIN, M.A., SHEPARD, T.H., & TANIMURA, T. (1972) A new in vitro culture technique for rat embryos. Teratology, 5: 367-376.

RODIER, P.M. (1976) Critical periods for behavioral anomalies in mice. Environm. Health Perspect., 18: 79-83.

RODIER, P.M. (1978) Behavioural teratology. In: Wilson, J.G. & Fraser, F.C., ed. Handbook of teratology, New York, London, Plenum Press, Vol. 4, pp. 397-428.

RODIER, P.M., REYNOLDS, S.S., & ROBERTS, W.N. (1979) Behavioral consequences of interference with CNS development in the early fetal period. Teratology, 19: 327-336.

ROSCHLAU, G. & JUSTUS, J. (1971) [Carcinogenic action of methotrexate and cyclophosphamide in ammrial experiments.] Dtsch. Gesundheitsw., 26: 219-222 (in German).

ROSENGARTEN, H. & FRIEDHOFF, A.J. (1979) Enduring changes in dopamine receptor cells of pups from drug administration to pregnant and nursing rats. Science, 203: 1133-1135.

RUCH, J.V. & KARCHER-DJURICIC, V. (1971) Action de la 5-fluoro-deoxyuridine sur la différenciation in vitro de molaires d'embryons de souris. Arch. biol., 82: 115-129.

RUNNER, M.N. (1965) Transplantation of mammalian ova: blastocyst and earlier stages. In: Wilson, J.G. & Warkany, J., ed. Teratology: principles and techniques, Chicago, London, The Univ. of Chicago Press, pp., 104-111.

RUSSELL, W.M.S. & BURCH, R.L. (1959) The principles of human experimental technique, London, Metheun, 238 pp.

RUSTIA, M. & SHUBIK, P. (1976) Transplacental effects of diethylstilbestrol on the genital tract of hamster offspring. Cancer Lett., 1: 139-146.

ŠABAD, L. M., KOLESNICHENKO, T. S., & SAVLUCHINSKAYA, L. A. (1973) Transplacental effect of carcinolipin in mice. Neoplasma, 20: 347-348.

SADLER, T.W. (1979a) Culture of early somite mouse embryos during organogenesis. J. Embryol. exp. Morphol., 49: 17-25.

SADLER, T.W. (1979b) Effects of hyperglycemic and diabetic rat serum on neural tube closure in early somite mouse embryos maintained in whole embryo culture. Anat. Rec., 193: 672 (abstract).

SALGANIK, R.I., GRYAZNOVA, I.M., MARKEL, A.L., MANANKOVA, N.M., & SOLOBYEVA, N.A. (1980) Enzymic "imprinting" as the result of early postnatal administration of enzyme inducers to animals. Exper. Basel, 36: 43-45.

SAXEN, I. (1965) Ontogenesis of virus resistance. In: Bergstrand, H. & Hellström, K.E., ed. Symposium on Virus and Cancer, Unio Nordica Contra Cancrum, Stockholm, Tryckeri Balder AB, pp. 150-161.

SAXEN, L. (1966) Effect of tetracycline on osteogenesis in vitro. J. exp. Zool., 162: 269-294.

SAXEN, I. (1973) Effects of hydrocortisone on the development in vitro of secondary palate in two inbred strains of mice. Arch. Oral Biol., 18: 1469-1479.

SAXEN, L. & EKBLOM, P. (1981) The developing kidney as a model system for normal and impaired organogenesis. In: Neubert, D. & Merker, H.-J., ed. Culture techniques. Applicability for studies on prenatal differentiation and toxicity, Berlin, New York, Walter de Gruyter Publ., pp. 291-300.

SAXEN, L. & KAITILA, I. (1972) The effect and mode of action of tetracycline on bone development in vitro. In: Klingberg, M.A., Abramovic, A., & Ckhemke, J., ed. Drugs and fetal development, New York, London, Plenum Press, pp. 205-218.

SAXEN, L. & LEHTONEN, E. (1978) Transfilter induction of kidney tubules as a function of the extent and duration of intercellular contacts. J. Embryol. exp. Morphol., 47: 97-109.

SAXEN, I. & SAXEN, L. (1975) Organ culture in teratology: Closure of the palatal shelves as a model system. In: Neubert, D. & Merker, H.-J., ed. New approaches to the evaluation of abnormal embryonic development, Stuttgart, Georg Thieme Publ., pp. 84-98.

SAXEN, L., KOSKIMIES, O., LAHTI, A., MIETTINEN, H., RAPOLA, J., & WARTIOVAARA, J. (1968) Differentiation of kidney mesenchyme in an experimental model system. Adv. Morphol., 7: 251-293.

SCANDALIOS, J.G. (1979) Physiological genetics, New York, Academic Press.

SCHACTER, L.P. (1970) Effect of conditioned media on differentiation in mass cultures of chick limb bud cells. I. Morphological effects. Ext. Cell Res., 63: 19-32.

SCHARDEIN, J.L. (1976) Drugs as teratogens, Cleveland, CRC Press.

SCHARDEIN, J.L. (1983) Teratogenic risk assessment - past, present, and future. In: Kalter, H., ed. Issues and reviews in teratology, New York, Plenum Publishing Corporation, pp. 181-214.

SCHNEIDER, J., WARZOK, R., OSSKE, G., & LEHNGUTH, CH. (1977a) [Tumor induction by various endogenously formed

N-nitroso ureas in the rat.] Zbl. allg. Pathol. u. pathol. Anat., 121: 61-75 (in German).

SCHNEIDER, J., WARZOK, R., & SCHWARZ, H. (1977b) [Endogenous formation of carcinogenic N-nitroso compounds in rats after application of drugs and nitrite.] Exp. Pathol. (Jena), 13(1): 32-43 (in German).

SCHNEIDER, J., WARZOK, R., SCHREIBER, D., & HEIDERSTADT, R. (1978) [Postnatal and transplacental carcinogenic action of methylmethane sulfonate (MMS) and ethylmethane sulfonate (EMS) in hooded rats.] Exp. Pathol. (Jena), 16(1/6): 157-167 (in German).

SCHOENTAL, R. & CAVANAGH, J. B. (1972) Brain and spinal cord tumors in rats treated with pyrrolizidine alkaloids. J. Natl Cancer Inst., 49(3): 665-671.

SCHREIWEIS, D.O. & MURRAY, G.J. (1976) Cardiovascular malformations in Oryzias latipes embryos treated with 2,4,5-trichlorophenoxyacetic acid (2,4,5-T). Teratology, 14: 287-290.

SCHULTZ, T.W., DUMONT, J.N., CLARK, B.R., & BUCHANAN, M.V. (1982) Embryotoxic and teratogenic effects of aqueous extracts of tar from coal gasification electrostatic precipitator. Teratog. Carcinog. Mutag., 2: 1-11.

SEHGAL, C.B. & HUTTON, J.J. (1977) Homogenates of pregnant rat and fetal tissues metabolize carcinogens to mutagens detected by Salmonella typhimurium TA98 and TA100. Mutat. Res., 46: 325-344.

SEIBEL, W. (1974) An ultrastructural comparison of the uptake and transport of horseradish peroxidase by the rat visceral yolk sac placenta during mid- and late gestation. Am. J. Anat., 140: 213-236.

SHENDRIKOVA, I.A. & ALEXANDROV, V.A. (1978) [Transplacental passage and carcinogenic action of nitrosodimethylamine in rats.] In: Conference on Carcinogenic N-nitrosocompounds - action, formation, detection. Tallin, pp. 89-90 (in Russian).

SHEPARD, T.H. (1965) The thyroid. In: De Haan, R.L. & Ursprung, H., ed. Organogenesis, New York, Holt, Rinehart and Winston, pp. 493-512.

SHEPARD, T.H. (1967) Onset of function in the human fetal thyroid: Biochemical and radioautographic studies from organ culture. J. clin. Endocrin., 27: 945-958.

SHEPARD, T.H. (1974) Embryonic and fetal thyroid development. In: Kelley, V., ed. Endocrine and metabolic disorders in children, Harper and Row, pp. 375-382.

SHEPARD, T.H. (1983) Catalog of teratogenic agents, 4th edition, Baltimore, London, Johns Hopkins University Press.

SHEPARD, T.H. & BASS, G.L. (1970) Organ culture of limb buds from riboflavin-deficient and normal rat embryos in normal and riboflavin-deficient media. Teratology, 3: 163-168.

SHEPARD, T.H. & FANTEL, A.G. (1981) Teratology of therapeutic agents. In: Iffy, L. & Kaminetzky, H.A., ed. Principles and practice of obstetrics and perinatology, New York, Wiley, J. and Sons, pp. 461-481.

SHEPARD, T.H., TANIMURA, T., & ROBKIN, M. (1969) In vitro study of rat embryos. I. Effects of decreased oxygen on embryonic heart rate. Teratology, 2: 107-110.

SHEPARD, T.H., TANIMURA, T., & ROBKIN, M.A. (1970) Energy metabolism in early mammalian embryos. Dev. Biol., Suppl. 4: 42-58.

SHEPARD, T.H., MILLER, J.R., & MAROIS, M., ed. (1975) Methods for Detection of Environmental Agents that Produce Congenital Defects, Amsterdam, Oxford, North-Holland Publ. Comp., New York, American Elsevier Publ. Comp. Inc., 263 pp.

SHEPARD, T.H., FANTEL, A.G., MIRKES, P.E., GREENAWAY, J.C., FAUSTMAN-WATTS, E., CAMPBELL, M., & JUCHAU, M.R. (in press) I. Teratology testing development and status of short-term prescreens. II. Biotransformation of teratogens as studied in whole embryo culture. In: Developmental Pharmacology.

SHIRLEY, E.A.C. & HICKLING, R. (1981) An evaluation of some statistical methods for analysing numbers of abnormalities found amongst litters in teratology studies. Biometrics, 37: 819-829.

SIEBER, S.M., & FABRO, S. (1971) Identification of drugs in the preimplantation blastocyst and in the plasma, uterine secretion and urine of the pregnant rabbit. J. Pharm. exp. Ther., 176: 65-75.

SIITERI, P.K. & WILSON, J.D. (1974) Testosterone formation and metabolism during male sexual differentiation in the human embryo. J. clin. Endocrinol. Metab., 38: 113-125.

SILANO, V., AURICCHIO, S., DE RITIS, G., DE VINCENZI, M., & OCCORSIO, P. (1981) Effects of gliadin-derived peptides from bread and durum wheat on small intestine cultures from rat fetus and coeliac children. In: Neubert, D. & Merker, H.-J., ed. Culture techniques. Applicability for studies on prenatal differentiation and toxicity, Berlin, New York, Walter de Gruyter Publ., pp. 385-394.

SMART, J.L. & DOBBING, J. (1971) Vulnerability of developing brain. II. Effects of early nutritional deprivation on reflex ontogeny and development of behaviour in the rat. Brain Res., 28: 85-95.

SMITH, M.K., KIMMEL, G., KOCHHAR, D., SHEPERD, T.H., STIELBERG, S., & WILSON, J. (in press) Selection of chemical compounds for in vitro teratogen test validation. Teratog. Carcinog. Mutag., __: -

SMITHBERG, M. (1962) Teratogenic effects of tolbutamide on the early development of the fish, Oryzias latipes. Am. J. Anat., 110: 205-213.

SNEDECOR, G.W. & COCHRAN, W.G. (1967) Statistical methods, 6th Edition, Ames, Iowa, Iowa State University Press, pp. 324-329.

SNOW, M.H.L. (1973) Abnormal development of pre-implantation mouse embryos grown in vitro with $^3$H-thymidine. J. Embryol. exp. Morph., 29: 601-615.

SNOW, M.H.L. (1975) The functional competence of the inner cell mass. In: Neubert, D. & Merker, H.-J., ed. New approaches to the evaluation of abnormal embryonic development, Stuttgart, Georg Thieme Publ., pp. 394-407.

SOBOTKA, T.J., COOK, M.P., & BRODIE, R.E. (1974) Effects of perinatal exposure to methylmercury on functional brain development and neurochemistry. Biol. Psychiat., 8: 307-320.

SOBRIAN, S.K. (1977) Prenatal morphine administration alters behavioural development in the rat. Biochem. Behav., 7: 285-288.

SOKAL, J.E. & LESSMANN, E.M. (1960) Effects of cancer chemotherapeutic agents on the human fetus. J. Am. Med. Assoc., 172: 1765-1771.

SOKAL, R. R. & ROHLF, F. J. (1969) Biometry. Assumptions of the analysis of variance, San Francisco, Freeman, pp. 367-402.

SOLURSH, M., AHRENS, P.B., & REITER, R.S. (1978) A tissue culture analysis of the steps in limb chondrogenesis. In Vitro, 14: 51-61.

SOTOMAYOR, R.E. & CUMMING, R.B. (1975) Induction of translocations by cyclophosphamide in different germ cell stages in male mice: cytological characterization and transmission. Mutat. Res., 27: 375-388.

SPATZ, M. & LAQUEUR, G.L. (1967) Transplacental induction of tumours in Sprague-Dawley rats with crude cycad material. J. Natl Cancer. Inst., 38: 233-245.

SPIELMANN, H. & EIBS, H.-G. (1977) Preimplantation embryos. Part I: Laboratory equipment, preparation of media, sampling and handling of the embryos. In: Neubert, D, Merker, H.-J., & Kwasigroch, T.E., ed. Methods in prenatal toxicology, Stuttgart, Georg Thieme Publ., pp. 210-220.

SPIELMANN, H., HABENICHT, U., EIBS, H.-G., JACOB-MÜLLER, U., & SCHIMMEL, A. (1981) Investigations on the mechanism of action and on the pharmacokinetics of cyclophosphamide treatment during the preimplantation period in the mouse. In: Neubert, D. & Merker, H.-J., ed. Culture techniques. Applicability for studies on prenatal differentiation and toxicity, Berlin, New York, Walter de Gruyter Publ., pp. 435-445.

SPYKER, D.A. & SPYKER, J.M. (1977) Response model analysis for cross-fostering studies: prenatal versus postnatal effects on offspring exposed to methylmercury dicyandiamide. Toxicol. appl. Pharmacol., 40: 511-527.

SPYKER, J.M. (1975) Assessing the impact of low level chemicals on development: behavioral and latent effects. Fed. Proc., 34: 1835-1844.

SPYKER, J.M. & FERNANDES, G. (1973) Impaired immune function in offspring from methylmercury treated mice. Teratology, 7: A28.

SPYKER, J.M., SPARBER, S.B., & GOLDBERG, A.M. (1972) Subtle consequences of methylmercury exposure: behavioral deviations in offspring of treated mothers. Science, 177: 621-623.

STAHLMANN, R., BLUTH, U., & NEUBERT, D. (1981) Effects of some "indirectly" alkylating agents on differentiation of limb buds in organ culture. In: Neubert, D. & Merker, H.-J., ed. Culture techniques. Applicability for studies on prenatal differentiation and toxicity, Berlin, New York, Walter de Gruyter Publ., pp. 207-221.

STAPLES, R.E. & HASEMAN, J.K. (1974) Selection of appropriate experimental units in teratology. Teratology, 9(3): 259-260.

STAVE, U. (1975) Perinatal changes of interorgan differences in cell metabolism. Biol. Neonat., 26: 318-332.

STAVROU, D. & LÜBBE, I., (1974) [Transplacental induction of kidney tumours in rabbits by ethylnitrososourea.] Verh. Dtsch. Ges. Path., 58: 545 (in German).

STAVROU, D., DAHME, E., & SCHRÖDER, B. (1977) [Transplacental neuro-oncogenic effect of ethylnitroso urea in rabbits during early embryogenesis.] Z. Krebsforsch., 89: 331-339 (in German).

STEBBINS, W.C. & RUDY, M.C. (1978) Behavioral ototoxicology. Environ. Health Perspect., 26: 43-51.

STEPTOE, P.C. & EDWARDS, R.G. (1978) Birth after the reimplantation of a human embryo. Lancet, II: 366.

STEVENS, L.C. (1967) The biology of teratomas. Adv. Morphog., 6: 1-31.

STREISINGER, G. (1975) Invited discussion. On the possible use of zebra fish for the screening of teratogens. In: Shepard, T.H., Miller, J.R., & Marois, M., ed. Methods for detection of environmental agents that produce congenital defects, Amsterdam, Oxford, New York, North-Holland Publ., pp. 59-64.

TABACOVA, S. (1983) Behavioural effects of prenatal exposure to nitrogen dioxide. 11th Conference of European Teratology Society, Paris, 29-31 August 1983 (abstracts).

TABACOVA, S., HINKOVA, L., NIKIFOROV, B., & BALABAEVA, L. (1981) Hazards for the progeny after maternal exposure to low carbon disulphide concentrations. G. Ital. med. Lav., 3: 121-125.

TANIMURA, T. (1980) Introductory remarks on behavioural teratology. Cong. Anom. 20: 301-318.

TESH, J.M. (1977) An approach to the assessment of postnatal development in laboratory animals. In: Neubert, D., Merker, H.-J., & Kwasigroch, T.E., ed. Methods in prenatal toxicology, Stuttgart, Georg Theime Publ., pp. 186-195.

THESLEFF, I. & PRATT, R.M. (1980) Tunicamycin inhibits mouse tooth morphogenesis and odontoblast differentiation in vitro. J. Embryol. exp. Morphol., 195-208.

THOMAS, J.B. (1968) Introduction to human embryology, Philadelphia, Lea & Febigert, 348 pp.

THORNTON, C.S. (1968) Amphibian limb regeneration. Adv. Morphog., 7: 205-249.

THORPE, E. (1967) Some pathological effects of hexachlorophene in the rat. J. comp. Pathol., 77: 137-142.

TILSON, H. & MITCHELL, C. (1980) Models for neurotoxicity. In: Hodgson, E., Bend, J., & Philpot, R., ed. Reviews in biomedical toxicology, New York, Elsevier, North Holland, pp. 265-294.

TILSON, H.A. & CABE. P.A. (1978) Strategy for the assessment of neurobehavioural consequences of environmental factors. Environ. Health Perspect., 26: 287-299.

TILSON, H., MITCHELL, O., & CABE, P. (1979) Screening for neurobehavioural toxicity: the need for and examples of validation of testing procedures. Neurobehav. Toxicol., 1 (Suppl.),: 137-148.

TILSON, H., CABE, P., & BURNE, T. (1980) Behavioural procedures for the assessment of neurotoxicity. In: Spencer, P.S. & Schaumburg, H.H., ed. Experimental and clinical neurotoxicology, Baltimore, Maryland, the Williams and Wilkins Co., pp. 758-766.

TOMATIS, L. (1979) Prenatal exposure to chemical carcinogens and its effect on subsequent generations. In: Prenatal carcinogenesis, Natl Cancer Inst. Monogr., 51: 159-184.

TOMATIS, L. & MOHR, U., ed. (1973) Transplacental Carcinogenesis, Lyon, IARC Sci. Publ., No. 4.

TOMATIS, L., CABRAL, J.R.P., LIKHACHEV, A.J., & PONOMARKOV, V. (1981) Increased cancer incidence in the progeny of male rats exposed to ethylnitrosourea before mating. Int. J. Cancer, 28: 475-478.

TROWELL, O.A. (1961) Problems in the maintenance of mature organs in vitro. In: La culture organotypique, Paris, Editions du Centre National de la Recherche Scientifique, pp. 237-249.

TSONIS, P.A. & EGUCHI, G. (1980) Teratogenic effects of carcinogens on limb regeneration in adult newts. Dev. Growth Differ., 22: 708 (abstract).

TURUSOV, V.S., ed. (1979) Pathology of tumours in laboratory animals, Vol. 2: Tumours of the mouse, Lyons, International Agency for Cancer Research, 669 pp. (IARC Scientific Publications No. 23).

TURUSOV, V.S., ed. (1982) Pathology of tumours in laboratory animals, Vol. 3: Tumours of the hamster, Lyons, International Agency for Cancer Research (IARC Scientific Publications No. 34).

TURUSOV, V.S., CHESTERMAN, F.C., DELLA PORTA, G., HOLLANDER, C.F., MOHR, U., ŠABAD, L.M., SOBIN, L.H., STANTON, M.F. & DAVIS, W., ed. (1973) Pathology of tumours in laboratory animals, Vol. 1: Tumours of the rat, Part 1, Lyons, International Agency for Cancer Research, 201 pp. (IARC Scientific Publications No. 5).

TURUSOV, V.S., CHESTERMAN, F.C., DELLA PORTA, G., HOLLANDER, C.F., MOHR, U., ŠABAD, L.M., SOBIN, L.H., STANTON, M.F. & (1976) Pathology of tumours in laboratory animals, Vol. 1: Tumours of the rat, Part 2, Lyons, International Agency for Cancer Research, 315 pp. (IARC Scientific Publications No. 5).

TYLER, A. & TYLER, B.S. (1966) The gametes; some procedures and properties. Physiology of fertilization and early development. In: Bvolootian, R.A., ed. Physiology of echinoderma, New York, Willy, I. & Sons Inc., Interscience Publ., pp. 639-741.

UMANSKY, R. (1966) The effect of cell population density on the developmental fate of reaggregating mouse limb bud mesenchyme. Dev. Biol., 13: 31-56.

US EPA (1980) Environmental Protection Agency, Mutagenicity risk assessment: proposed guidelines. Fed. Reg., 45(221): 74984-74988.

US EPA (1982) Environmental Protection Agency, Assessment of risk to human reproductive system and to development of the human conceptus from exposure to environment substances. In: Proceedings of the US EPA sponsored conference, Oakridge, Tennessee, Oakridge National Laboratory, 1982. Springfield, Virginia, National Technical Information Service (NTIS No. DE 82-007897).

US EPA (1975) Environmental Protection Agency. Pesticide programs. Registration, re-registration, and classification procedures. Fed. Reg., 40: 28242-28286.

US EPA (1976) Environmental Protection Agency. Health risk and economic impact assessments of suspected carcinogens. Interim procedures and guidelines. Fed. Reg., 41: 21402-21405.

US EPA (1978) Environmental Protection Agency, chemical substances inventory (Cumulative supplement (TS-799), July).

VERGIEVA, T. (1981) [Teratogenicity and embryotoxicity]. In: Kaloyanova, F., ed. Hygienna Toksikologia. Med. i Fizkul. (Sofia), pp. 148-155 (in Bulgarian).

VERGIEVA, T. (1982) [Karbendazim: teratogenic effects in rats]. Hig. Zdr., 4: 333-339 (in Bulgarian).

VERGIEVA, T., ZAJKOV, CH., & ANTOV, G. (1981a) [Prenatal alcohol exposure-changes in behaviour and activity of some brain enzymes.] Hig. Zdr., 6: 532-537 (in Bulgarian).

VESSELINOVITCH, S.D. (1973) Comparative studies on prenatal carcinogenesis. In: Tomatis, L., Mohr, U., & Davis, W., ed. Transplacental carcinogenesis, Lyons, International Agency for Cancer Research, pp. 14-22 (IARC Scientific Publications No. 4).

VESSELINOVITCH, S.D. & RAO, K.V.N. (1974) Transplacental and neonatal carcinogenesis experimental approach. In: Characterization of human tumours, Amsterdam, New York, Elsevier, pp. 135-150.

VESSELINOVITCH, S.D., RAO, K.V.N., & MIHAILOVICH, N. (1979) Neoplastic response of mouse tissues during perinatal age periods and its significance in chemical carcinogenesis. In: Perinatal carcinogenesis. Natl Cancer Inst. Monogr., 51: 239-250.

VITVITSKAYA, B.R., SAVONICHEVA, G.A., SEMENOVA, A.A., & SKACHKOVA, V.N. (1980) [Hygienic evaluation of the major components of waste water from the production of antimicrobial materials.] Hig. i. Sanit., 10: 70-73 (in Russian).

VORHEES, C.V., BRUNNER, R.L., & BUTCHER, R.E. (1979) Psychotropic drugs as behavioural teratogens. Science, 205: 1220-1225.

VOUK, V.B. & SHEEHAN, P.J. (1983) Methods for assessing the effects of chemicals on reproductive functions, Chichester, Sussex, England, John Wiley & Sons, 480 pp.

WARTIOVAARA, J., NORDLING, S., LEHTONEN, E., & SAXEN, L. (1974) Transfilter induction of kidney tubules: correlation with cytoplasmic penetration into nuclepore filters. J. Embryol. exp. Morphol., 31: 667-682.

WATANABE, N. (1979) Environmental determinants of birth defects prevalence. In: Klingberg, M.A., Weatherall, J.A.C., ed. Epidemiological methods for detection of teratogens, Contributions to epidemiology and biostatistics, Basel, Munchen, Paris, London, New York, Sidney, Karger, S., pp. 91-100.

WEIL, C.S. (1970) Selection of the valid number of sampling units and a consideration of their combination in toxicological studies involving reproduction, teratogenesis, or carcinogenesis. Food Cosmet. Toxicol., 8: 177-182.

WEIL, C.S. (1972) Guidelines for experiments to predict the degree of safety of a material for man. Toxicol. appl. Pharmacol., 21: 194-199.

WEISS, B. (1975) Effects on behaviour. In: Principles for evaluating chemicals in the environment, Washington, DC, National Academy of Sciences National Research Council, pp. 198-216.

WELCH, R.M., HARRISON, Y.E., GOMMI, B.W., POPPERS, P.J., FINSTER, M., & CONNEY, A.H. (1969) Stimulatory effect of cigarette smoking on the hydroxylation of 3,4-benzpyrene and the N-dimethylation of 3-methyl-4-monomethylaminoazobenzene by enzymes in human placenta. Clin. Pharmacol. Ther., 10: 100-109.

WELSCH, F., BAUMANN, I., & NEUBERT, D. (1978) Effects of methyl-parathion and methyl-paraoxon on morphogenetic differentiation of mouse limb buds in organ culture. In: Neubert, D., Merker, H.-J., Nau, H., & Langman, J., ed. Role of pharmacokinetics in prenatal and perinatal toxicology, Stuttgart, Georg Thieme Publ., pp. 351-358.

WERBOFF, J., GOTTLIEB, J.S., HAVLENA, J., & WORD, T.J. (1961) Behavioural effects of prenatal drug administration in the white rat. Pediatrics, 27: 318-324.

WERBOFF, J., HAVLENA, J., & SIKOV, M.R. (1962) Effects of prenatal X-irradiation on activity, emotionality and maze-learning ability in the rat. Radiat. Res., 16: 441-452.

WHITTEN, W.K. (1971) Nutrient requirements for the culture of preimplantation embryos in vitro. In: Raspé, G., ed. Advances in the biosciences, Oxford - Braunschweig, Pergamon Press - Vieweg, Vol. 6, pp. 129-141.

WHITTINGHAM, D.G. (1971) Culture of mouse ova. J. Reprod. Fertil. Suppl., 14: 7-21.

WHO (1967) Principles for the Testing of Drugs for Teratogenicity, World Health Organization, Geneva, 18 pp. (WHO Technical Reports Series No. 364).

WHO (1978) Principles and Methods for Evaluating the Toxicity of Chemicals, Part 1, World Health Organization, Geneva, p. 19 (Environmental Health Criteria No. 6).

WILSON, J.G. (1965) Methods for administering agents and detecting malformations in experimental animals. In: Wilson, J.G. & Warkany, J., ed. Teratology: Principles and techniques, Chicago, University of Chicago Press, pp. 262-277.

WILSON, J.G. (1973a) Environment and birth defects, New York, San Francisco, London, Academic Press, p. 180.

WILSON, J.G. (1977) Current status of teratology. General principles and mechanisms derived from animal studies. In: Wilson, J.G. & Fraser, F.C., ed. Handbook of teratology: General principles and etiology, New York, Plenum Press, Vol. 1, pp. 47-74.

WILSON, J.G. (1978a) Survey of in vitro systems: Their potential use in teratogenicity screening. In: Wilson, J.G. & Fraser, F.C., ed. Handbook of teratology, New York, London, Plenum Press, Vol. 4, pp. 135-153.

WILSON, J.G. (1978b) Review of _in vitro_ systems with potential for use in teratogenicity screening. _J. environ. Pathol. Toxicol._, _2_: 149-167.

WILSON, J.G. & FRASER, F.C., ed. (1977) _Handbook of teratology_, New York, London, Plenum Press, Vol. 1, 1476 pp.

WOO, D.C. & HOAR, R.M. (1979) Reproductive performance and spontaneous malformations in control Charles River CD rats: A joint study by MARTA. In: _Annual Meeting of Teratology Society_.

WOO, D.C. & HOAR, R.M. (1982) Reproductive performance and spontaneous malformations in control New Zealand White rabbits: A joint study by Middle Atlantic Reproduction and Teratology Association. In: _Annual meeting of Teratology Society_.

YANAL, J. (1979) Long-term induction of microsomal drug oxidizing system in mice following prenatal exposure to barbiturate. _Biochem. Pharmacol._, _28_: 1429-1430.

ZBINDEN, G. (1981) Experimental methods in behavioral teratology. _Arch. Toxicol._, _48_: 69-88.

ZELLER, W.J. (1980) [Prenatal carcinogenic action of 5-(3,3-dimethyl-1-triazeno)-imidazol-4-carboxamide (DTIC) on the offspring of BD 1X Rats.] _Arch. Geschwulstforsch._, _50_: 306-308 (in German).